SHAMANISM
WITHOUT BORDERS

A Guide to Shamanic Tending for Trauma and Disasters

A Society for
Shamanic Practitioners
Handbook

Society for Shamanic Practitioners

2300 Eighth Street, Olivenhain, CA USA 92024
760-586-8252
www.shamansociety.org

Copyright © 2011 Society for Shamanic Practitioners
All Rights Reserved. Published 2011

No portion of this book may be reproduced in whole or in part, by any means (with the exception of short quotes for the purpose of review), without permission of the publisher. Printed in the United States of America on recycled paper using soy-based ink

11   10   09   08   07   06   05   1   2   3   4   5   6   7

ISBN: 978-0-615-41710-3

Edited by Bonnie Horrigan
Designed by Ron Short

Contributors

"First Thoughts" © 2010 by Cecile Carson, MD, Tom Cowan, PhD, and Bonnie Horrigan

"Historical Perspectives" © 2010 by Sandra Ingerman, MA, and José Stevens, PhD

"Modern Perspectives on an Ancient Art: The Healing Location," "Healing at the Scene of an Accident" © 2010 by Jose Stevens, PhD

"Energetic Fields in the Landscape" © 2010 by Ana Larramendi

"Using Light and Positive Visualization" © 2010 by Sandra Ingerman, MA

"Shamanic Responses to Disaster" © 2010 by Carol Proudfoot-Edgar, CSC, and Cecile Carson, MD

"Ethical Considerations" © 2010 by Tom Cowan, PhD

"Working with Shelter Animals" © 2010 by Carol Proudfoot-Edgar, CSC

"Healing When Multiple Accidents Occur at the Same Place," "Finding Missing Persons" © 2010 by Pamela Albee

"The Star Gazer Shamanic Moon Bear Project: Brave Compassion" © 2010 by Lora Jansson

"Reflections from the 2010 SSP Conference" © 2010 by Tom Cowan, PhD, Bonnie Horrigan, Carol Proudfoot-Edgar, and José Stevens, PhD

"Final Points" © 2010 by Lena Stevens

All materials reprinted by permission of the authors.

In Appreciation

The Society for Shamanic Practitioners would like to thank the following for contributing content from their journey work for Haiti:

Lyn Birmingham
Jane Burns
Ramona Gault
Julie Lange Groth

Cover photography and design by Ron Short, Ron Short Studios, Santa Fe, NM

Contents

First Thoughts ~ 1

The Foundation

Historical Perspectives ~ 5

Modern Perspectives ~ 9

Energetic Fields in the Land ~ 13

Using Light and Positive Visualization ~ 17

Shamanism without Borders Guidelines

Shamanic Responses to Disasters ~ 23

Ethical Considerations ~ 27

The Practice

Working with Shelter Animals ~ 27

Healing at the Scene of an Accident ~ 39

Healing when Multiple Accidents Occur in the Same Place ~ 45

Finding Missing Persons ~ 47

The Shamanic Moon Bear Project ~ 51

Land-Tending at a Windmill Site ~ 61

Reflections from the SSP 2010 Conference ~ 65

Final Points ~ 75

The Society for Shamanic Practitioners ~ 79

About the Authors ~ 80

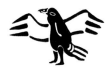

How to Read this Book

THIS HANDBOOK IS NOT A BLUEPRINT. Every disaster is different and each person, animal and place affected by an event needs to be diagnosed and worked with in a way that addresses the specific needs of the time and circumstances. It is important to journey and find the "individual medicine"— the healing ceremony, ritual, or process — that is right for the uniqueness of the situation. This book simply provides a collection of philosophies and possibilities that can form a solid foundation for the work. Practitioners should read between the lines and listen between the words for Spirit to speak and comment.

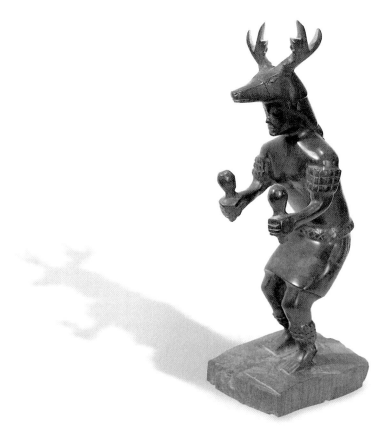

First Thoughts
Cecile Carson, MD, Tom Cowan, PhD and Bonnie Horrigan

THE IDEA OF SHAMANISM WITHOUT BORDERS has been rising in the consciousness of many shamanic practitioners for the past decade. We live in a troubled world in which terrorism, war, pollution, and natural disasters cause disruption and suffering to humanity, to the animal and plant life, and to the earth's delicate biosystem.

Our ability, through mass media, to instantly see disasters unfolding has heightened our awareness of these events across the globe. By simply turning on the TV or going on the Internet, we can "be there" — we can see the destruction earthquakes have caused in China, Chile, and Haiti; we can witness the flattened coastal towns in the aftermath of the tsunami in Japan; and we can watch a tornado tear apart a 10-mile stretch of land in Mississippi, laying waste to everything in its path. The invaluable presence of first responders is apparent. They find the missing, bury the dead, feed the hungry, and tend to what has been broken.

At the 2007 board meeting for the Society for Shamanic Practitioners (SSP) in Santa Fe, New Mexico, we asked ourselves if we, as shamanic practitioners, had anything of value to add to these rescue efforts? Our answer was yes; we thought we did. But we were not thinking we would duplicate the French organization Doctors Without Borders, which sends medical teams into disaster areas around the world. Instinctively, even though the vision was not yet clear, we felt a shamanic organization would look and operate very differently. Doctors Without Borders tends to the physical needs of people. It seemed to us that Shamanism Without Borders would tend to the energetic and spiritual wounds.

We held a Shamanism Without Borders "think tank" at the 2008 SSP conference to gather input from conference attendees. Then we further discussed how we could begin to manifest the project at the 2008 and 2009 board meetings. At the 2009 meeting, we decided to build a conference that would put our ideas to the test and consequently, our 2010 conference was dedicated solely to Shamanism Without Borders activities.

Opposite: Photomontage by Ron Short © 2010.

We believe that shamanic knowledge can assist people in tending to the suffering of land, animals, and people when a disaster occurs, and we feel strongly that a shamanic presence, whether physical or in spirit, can help those who find their "normal" life patterns seriously disrupted.

On a very primary level, the shaman's call is to provide hope and inspiration, compassion, comfort, and healing. The shaman is concerned with the soul's journey from birth through death and beyond. This concern is not only for the souls of humans, but the soul-filled manifestation of Spirit in all beings.

Certainly there are individuals and some groups of shamanic practitioners who already respond to such events. We each have various informal networks we write or call when a concern arises for which we solicit remote healing and prayers. And, in fact, we have included in this Handbook several accounts from people already engaged in this work. However, much of contemporary shamanism has focused on the individual needing healing with less attention given to the community itself or to the larger world.

The perceived needs can be overwhelming for one individual alone, whereas much benefit can be derived from the joint efforts of shamans. How can we transcend our individual lives and reach out through an organized group effort? How can we respond as a shamanic community? These are the questions that members of the Society for Shamanic Practitioners have been asking and this is the collective journey we have chosen to take.

In this time on the planet, we are called to combine what have been traditional shamanic responses to disasters with the direct guidance of Spirit to forge new ways to help the global community and the planet itself. Welcome to the journey.

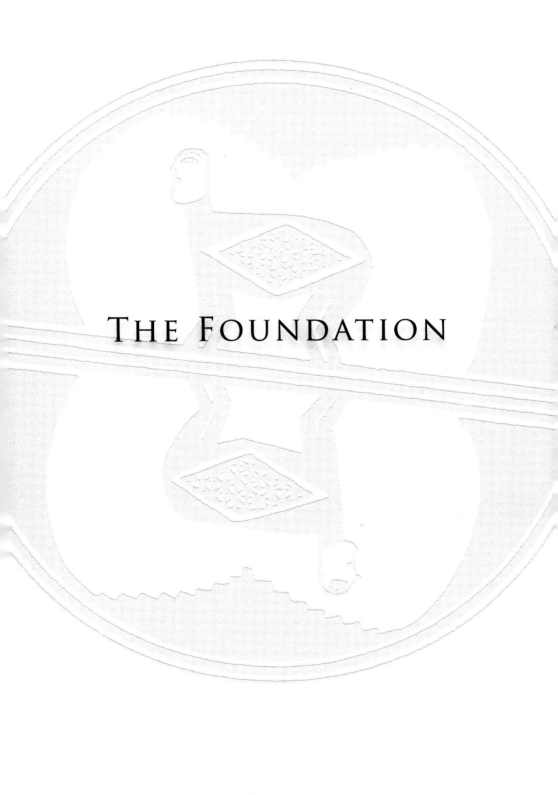

THE FOUNDATION

Historical Perspectives
Sandra Ingerman, MA, and José Stevens, PhD

Traditionally, shamans have always helped the people in their communities cope with disasters that occur, whether it was an incident of contagious illness, natural disasters such as earthquakes or volcanic eruptions, war, or human-caused pollution.

Soul Retrieval

Most shamanic cultures understand that illness has a spiritual cause and performing soul retrievals is a core method of healing for both people and the land.

In diagnosing soul loss for land, practitioners should be careful to not anthropomorphize the incident. Numerous environmental events, which humans might label a catastrophe or trauma, are actually natural processes of healing and evolution for the earth. For example, forest fires are traumatic to the people and animals who have lost their homes or who have been hurt, but the earth needs forest fires to regenerate herself. Many of the seeds that birth into trees and plants require the heat of fire to germinate.

In order to learn what is needed, practitioners must journey to their helping spirits for a diagnosis to determine if healing is even necessary. It is equally important to check with one's helping spirits to receive information before conducting soul retrievals for the people and animals involved.

Psychopomp Work

When a disaster has caused human death there is the possibility that some of the souls of the deceased might get stuck in the Middle World and not move on to a transcendent reality. The shock of the disaster can create confusion and the newly dead might not understand they have died, or they may want to stay close to be of help to loved ones, or they may be disoriented and can't find their way out of the Middle World.

It has always been the role of the shaman to perform psychopomp work. The shaman leads souls who are stuck in the Middle World into the transcendent worlds. There are documented psychopomp ceremonies for individuals and small groups and also ceremonies to lead mass groups of people into the loving arms of the universe.

In her experience as a shamanic teacher, Sandra Ingerman has witnessed spirits creating a vortex or light column through which mass numbers of souls were led by the light into a transcendent world. She experienced this in the massacre in Luxor, Egypt in the late 1990's as well as with the tragedy of September 11, 2001 in the United States and the earthquakes in China and Haiti.

The key in working with psychopomp ceremonies involving the crossing over of souls is to make sure you are filled with power. It is not uncommon for a lost and confused soul to possess a practitioner or witnesses to such a ceremony. Everyone present must be filled with power so there are no empty spaces for the lost souls to fill. Psychopomp work, like soul retrievals, can help heal trauma in people, animals, and the land.

Ceremony

Shamans also perform a variety of other ceremonies to create balance and harmony between the people and the spirits of weather and those spirits that will keep balance in the environment. For instance, grieving ceremonies are performed to support members in the community who have lost homes or loved ones.

The Shipibos of the upper Amazon and the Huichol tribe of the Sierras in Central Mexico both perform ceremony to cleanse the land of lost spirits and invoke the powers of Spirit to restore balance. Additionally, both sing to the land to rejuvenate it. Each, however, employs some different techniques.

The Huichols make use of fire, the sacred god Tatawari, who represents the sun on earth, to cleanse the landscape and protect all from negativity. The Shipibo make liberal use of tobacco, another form of the spirit of fire in consort with a plant spirit, to clear and heal the environment. Both employ sacred water to cleanse the people and the land itself. In the case of the Shipibo, it is perfumed water infused with *icaros* or sacred songs. In the case of the Huichols, it is salt water from the sea infused with sacred songs.

Both cultures believe in the power of singing to the land. This wakes the land up, restores balance, and reconnects the land to the highest form of Spirit. Finally, both use the power of sacred breath to blow prayers, songs and healing onto people animals, and the landscape itself.

The Q'ero of the high Andes in Peru are one of the few carriers of the ancient pre-Incan traditions left. They live in an extremely challenging terrain between ten and sixteen thousand feet where many avalanches and rockfalls occur. They say that people and their environments may accumulate *hoocha*, non resonant energies that can cause imbalances and difficulties for both people, animals and the environments they live within. A person not cleansed of *hoocha* may draw to themselves an accident on the trail. *Hoocha* remaining on the trail may cause an accident for animals or other people. They are also quick to say that while this *hoocha* is not a bad thing in and of itself, it is simply not compatible with being healthy, happy and powerful. Therefore they have been given practices by the mountain spirits for removing this *hoocha* so that it does not linger to create problems for themselves or others.

They begin by making offerings to the land in the form of *despachos*, symbolic presents to the mountain spirits, offerings they burn after expressing many prayers of thanks for all they have been helped with. Then they use their mesas, personalized wrapped cloths containing objects of power, to remove the *hoocha* from the person or the place. In order not to leave a vacuum, they use their mesas to bring in *Sami*, starlight energy from the sky to replace the *hoocha*. They say that starlight is the highest frequency and is completely incompatible with *hoocha*. Starlight will only attract positive harmonious experiences. Starlight is what human beings are meant to thrive on, not *hoocha*. After completing this process, all is put back into balance once again. In this way they have learned to live with the mountains and its challenges.

Learning how to live a life of honor and respect for nature and the elements is key in creating harmony and balance. Learning simple ceremonies to create harmony and balance are essential for the times we live in.

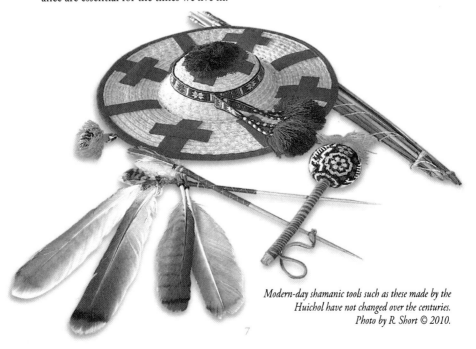

Modern-day shamanic tools such as these made by the Huichol have not changed over the centuries.
Photo by R. Short © 2010.

Modern Perspectives on an Ancient Art: The Healing of Location

José Stevens, PhD

SHAMANISM HAS ALWAYS BEEN A WAY for people to work with what we now call the quantum field. In the past, shamans did not have the scientific terminology of physics to discuss their insights and methods but nevertheless they were able to conduct their business with power and skill. Today we are able to integrate the cutting edge understandings of quantum physics and ancient shamanic techniques for a much fuller understanding of how shamans manipulate reality.

According to quantum physics all locations are merely collections of information in the form of light waves perceived as real by human beings. These collections of information have coherence but may lose some of their coherence due to the influence of other streams of information that bump into them, interface with them, or influence them. In other words, shamanically speaking, the assemblage point of the location may have been moved or jarred from its former position. Thus a village in a valley may be impacted by the intensity of death caused by an avalanche set off by a large local earthquake. The valley may no longer have the coherence it had before the earthquake and may now hold warped information that impacts people in harmful ways when they pass through there and interface with it. Shamans of old would have perceived this imbalance and set about performing a ceremony that would bring coherence back to the valley.

In order to accomplish this, they would have had to assess or diagnose the change in the pattern of the valley. They would then have to understand the most effective methods to clear out the non-resonant information by communicating with the various information sources in the area, that is spirits and guides. Based on this exchange they might embark on rebalancing the area (restoring the assemblage point) through singing, chanting, introducing sacred geometry, or numerous other methods. Since they knew their ability to observe the valley actually changed the valley, they knew they had to observe it in a

Opposite: José Stevens at Mount Quemado, Mexico. Photo by R. Short © 2010.

special way. This is an oversimplification but gives some idea how shamanic healing of a location can be understood in the cutting edge parlance of quantum physics.

In a similar way souls in successful transition can be seen as coherent bodies of information in transition or transformation. However some souls, due to their violent deaths, have lost their coherence and focus. Their assemblage points were shocked and moved violently without preparation. So these souls (standing waves who have lost their form) would need coherence restored so they can refocus and manifest where they need to be next.

This leads to a final point. One of the wonderful contributions of quantum physics is the ancient understanding that since everything is connected, a simple act of observation can initiate important changes in alignment with the values and intentions of the observer. Understanding this leads to the insight that to initiate powerful healing, very little needs to be done. After listening to Spirit carefully for instructions, a simple song or prayer, an offering of tobacco, a request for forgiveness or compassion may be all that is needed to set things right again. Since there is always much help in the spirit world, we need not do everything ourselves. Rather, much can be delegated to capable elementals, *poderios* (powers) and spirits willing to help. So with this understanding there is little need for struggle, efforting, or massive response. A little bit goes a long way.

Mapacho, rattle, feather, and mesas containing crystals, stones, and other sacred objects. Photo by R. Short © 2010.

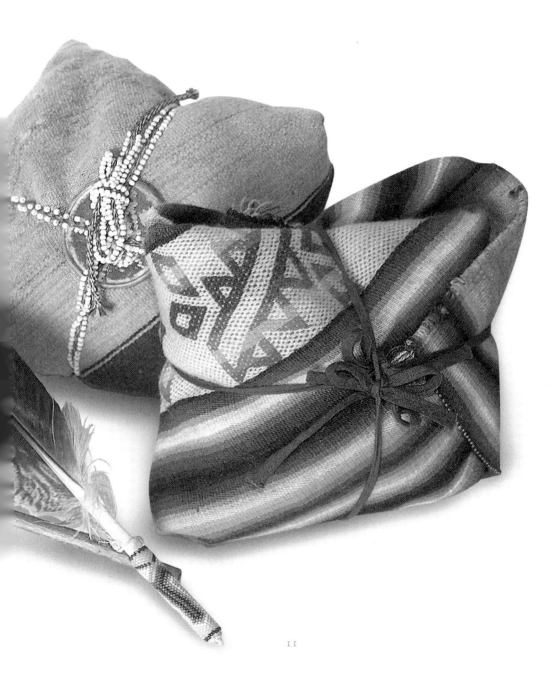

Energetic Fields in the Landscape

Ana Larramendi

As part of their healing work, Shamanism Without Borders practitioners engage in the restoration of energetic balance to the landscape. A knowledge base of the types of energetic fields that crisscross the world is therefore helpful.

Ley lines: Part of the matrix of geomagnetic lines that crisscross the surface of the earth, ley lines are naturally occurring channels on the earth that appear to be aligned to contours of the land, underground rivers, and places of power, as well as having orientation to stars, solstices, and equinoxes. They are the earth's meridians through which electromagnetic energy travels.

***Ceke* lines:** *Cekes* (a Peruvian Quechua word) are human-created geomagnetic lines and meridians used to establish an energetic connection to sacred sites, places of power (*huacas* and *pacarinas*) and places of high energy. *Ceke* lines at times overlap with ley lines. Shamans create *ceke* lines through intention, ritual, and invocation. In Quechua cosmology, all power places are interconnected by this web of *ceke* and ley lines, and are located where two or more of these lines intersect. *Cekes* stretch like a spider web over the land, and the shaman is like the spider who feels the vibration of the web. Shamans may create a *ceke* line to redirect a blocked ley line so the energy flow of the landscape is balanced, not unlike coronary bypass surgery.

***Huaca*:** A powerful place in the landscape where there is a convergence of *kausay*. In Quechua *kausay* is the vital living energy that animates the cosmos. This is similar to *prana* in Hindu or *chi* (qi) in Taoism. *Huacas* are located where *ceke* and ley lines intersect. These places draw energy from the landscape or sky. Locations of heightened power have long been recognized as places where the veils between the worlds are thin and access to the divine is heightened. Some of these places are natural — like cliffs, dramatic rock formations, mountains, or high promontories — others are made by humans. Their power has been enhanced by regular visitations and repeated use in ceremony to awaken the spirit of the landscape, as with sacred sites, burials, effigy mounds, cairns, temples, synagogues, and churches. Often sacred sites are built on *huacas* to intensify the spiritual powers of the site.

Pacarinas: A *pacarina* is Quechua for a creation place in the landscape. At *pacarinas* there is an emergence of *kausay* from the earth in springs, caves, waterfalls, and natural formations. Birth and creation energy have often been central to many shamanic cultures; the ritualizing of birth, death, rebirth and renewal has often been tied to caves and springs. Because of this connection there are many sacred and religious sites associated with *pacarinas*.

Vortexes: A vortex is a place where the energies of two or more *ceke* or ley lines converge or where a mineral deposit exists that creates the conditions of an energetic whirlpool. Vortexes are spherical fields of concentrated energy that flow in or out in the form of a torus (a three-dimensional doughnut-shaped surface) and originate from magnetic, spiritual, or other unknown sources. Additionally, vortexes can act as a portal between the spirit world and this world. Vortexes typically exist where there are strong concentrations of gravitational anomalies and can create the sensation of bending and shifting time or space due to a convergence of energy fields. Vortexes can be used to accelerate the healing and clearing of a place, or else to receive an abundance of energy.

Imprints: Imprints are energy fields created by an event or activity. Imprints can be positive if they affirm and revitalize life force. Labyrinths, gardens, landscapes, and even buildings that are created in a sustainable manner and with the guidance of nature spirits will create a life-affirming imprint on the land. Imprints can also manifest in a more negative form in places where repeated violence has occurred. The imprint can manifest as an overabundance of one particular element, as a site of frequent accidents, or as the deadening of a natural landscape.

Background: Labyrinth at Grace Cathedral in downtown San Francisco, California. Photo by Marlith © 2008 (GNU Free Documentation License).

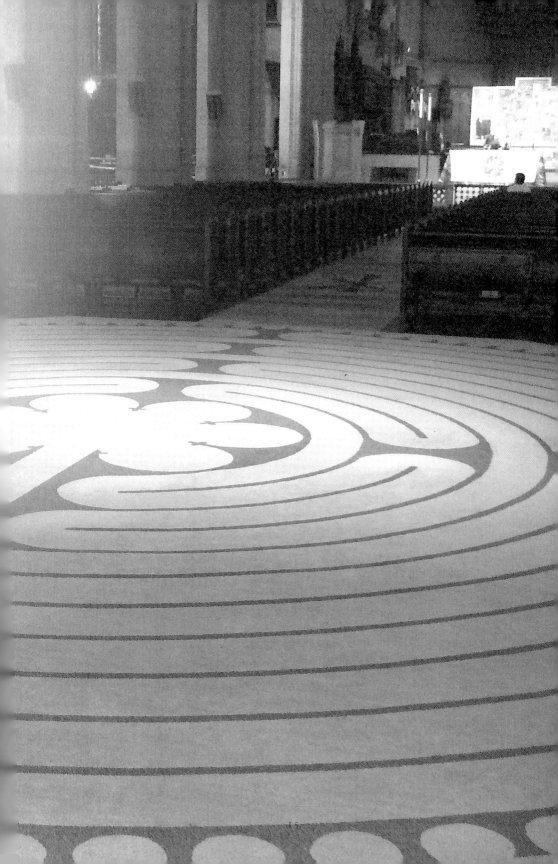

Using Light and Positive Visualization

Sandra Ingerman, MA

With journey insight from Julie Lange Groth

Numerous stories from shamanic cultures across the globe describe the great shamans as people who had a transcendent experience of light and oneness. It is through this experience that shamans gained their healing and clairvoyant abilities.

When we go within and experience ourselves as more than our body or our thoughts we find our inner core, which is pure spiritual light. The body and the mind clothe this light and when we are that spiritual light, we experience the unified field in which we are connected to the web of life.

As human beings, our experience contains a paradox. On one level we suffer from loss, illness and mental states such as fear and anger. On another level we are pure divine light that has nothing to lose and is one with the creative forces of the universe. One powerful way to work shamanically is to radiate light into the darkness that is experienced during a disaster. If everyone pities those who have experienced loss and trauma, that actually pushes the victims deeper into the hole. When we perceive people in their divine light and perfection, we feed their spiritual strength, which will help them to rise out of their situation. We want to feed the light instead of feeding the darkness.

While we should always have compassion for what people are going through, radiating light to the land, the people and animals will assist in creating a path that brings about healing and positive change. Additionally, when we work together as a global community, there is an exponential energy to create healing.

Years ago when Santa Fe was in a severe drought, I envisioned all the trees where I live in their divine light. I couldn't give them water but I could perceive them in their divinity. I have a camera called a GDV camera that takes photos of the energy fields of people and substances.

One of the trees on the land where I live is a peach tree and I brought one of its peaches to a Medicine for the Earth training in which I was teaching people how to use spiritual light to heal the environment. When we began the workshop we took a photo of the energy and life force of the peach. It looked good. That night we performed a ceremony where fifty of us experienced our divine light and perceived everyone and everything in our meeting space as divine light. Afterwards, using the same GDV camera we took a photo of the energy field of the peach. In that photo, the energy of the peach was so much more vibrant. This is a tangible example of the power of working in community.

When there is news of a disaster or environmental situation, it is important to open our hearts and experience compassion for the suffering that has occurred. At the same time don't feed the suffering. Quiet your mind, go within and state the intention: "Thank you for taking from me what keeps me separate from my divine light and perfection."

Experience your spiritual light and absorb this light into every cell of your being like a dry sponge absorbing water. Soak in it. Then radiate this light into the world while focusing your light on the area and people in need. (Notice that we do not send light or energy. We become spiritual light and, like a star, we radiate that light.)

The light will create a light column or vortex that will help the deceased transcend. The light will also stimulate the radiance of the land, people and animals to shine. The world we live in is simply a projection of our thoughts, words and imaginations. We can daydream a world of suffering or we can use our imaginations to create a world of peace, love, light, harmony, and abundance.

If you gather a group to do this work together, all the better. If you work alone, you can always join in with a global circle of thousands who do work in this way.

Here is an example of how Julie Lange Groth, a shamanic teacher, used this principle to work spiritually for Haiti after a devastating earthquake: "In my journey I saw a haze of light forming over Haiti, and within it the city of Port-au-Prince was already being rebuilt on the spiritual plane. It was clear we had the opportunity to join in the rebuilding by dreaming a new dream for Haiti. I asked my students to hold a vision of a Haiti in which there is no poverty, where everyone has a home, safety, food, education, healthcare, and stability. I also saw that in the new Haiti, the old ways were being reclaimed, and people were learning to live in harmony and balance with the elements and the land, so they were no longer so vulnerable to hurricanes, earthquakes and tsunamis.

"For the rescue workers who are physically there trying to help, there is no way to escape the devastation of what has happened. But as light-workers and dreamers, when we focus on the suffering, we feed the vision of a Haiti that continues to be devastated, poor, hungry, uneducated, and unstable. Instead, we can use our powers of imagination and visualization to feed the dream of a new Haiti, one in which everyone has a home, food, jobs, health care, education, and hope for the future."

Shamans teach that the world we live in is a dream, and many shamanic cultures are now sharing that we are living the wrong dream. It is our responsibility to learn how to dream a good dream and teach others how to do the same. This means putting yourself fully into the world you wish to live in, and using all your senses to build an invisible world of substance that creates the physical world. All spiritual traditions teach that everything begins in the invisible before it manifests in the physical.

See the colors and all the visuals of the place you are working with or for the planet itself in complete beauty and perfect health. Smell the fragrances of a healthy environment. Hear the sounds of laughter. Feel the joy of people and other life living in harmony. Taste the food that is filled with vibrant light and life force.

Don't watch the dream as if you are watching a movie or TV. Step into your dream and be part of it. Experience the dream as if it is happening now, not some time in the future. As you continue to work with your dreaming, start to focus on aligning your thoughts and words with the vision you are creating. This is an important daily practice.

All birth comes from within. A baby grows in a womb before being birthed into the outer world. Trees and plants begin as seeds that grow beneath the surface of the earth. Our world and all outer events start from an inner process in our inner landscape.

The key to working spiritually as an agent of conscious change is to learn to dream and align your thoughts and words with your desired outcome. Focus on what you want to create.

Many of us feel hopeless and powerless to help on the physical level, but we do have power to help in disasters and for the planet at large by engaging in spiritual practices in our daily lives and working together as a global community.

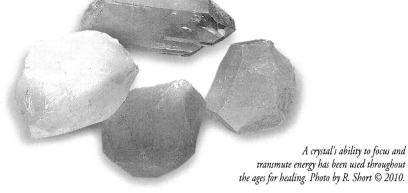

A crystal's ability to focus and transmute energy has been used throughout the ages for healing. Photo by R. Short © 2010.

Shamanism without Borders Guidelines

Shamanic Responses to Disasters

Carol Proudfoot-Edgar, CSC, and Cecile Carson, MD

THE SHAMANIC RESPONSE to any disaster should include the following steps:
- Assess the nature and extent of trauma
- Engage with the spirits and beings within the affected environment
- Create a team of helping spirits
- Identify the different healing approaches for working directly or remotely
- Develop a group that can be a 'response team'
- Apply specific healing methods appropriate to the place and space
- Employ ceremonies that support and bless the healing work involved
- Tend personal issues that arise in doing this work

Phases of Disaster Recovery

The recovery process naturally involves four stages of progressive healing.

Acute Phase – The acute phase is characterized by shock and intense emotional response and heroic behaviors. It involves the mobilization of shamanic responses: creating the team of spirit helpers, psychopomp and soul retrieval work, contact with spirits of the land involved, contact with weather spirits, networking with other shamanic practitioners, group ceremony, sharing experiences, and encouraging each other.

If visiting a site as a shamanic response team, practitioners should support beings affected by the disaster as well as human relief-workers on site, and coordinate knowledge with these workers as appropriate (e.g. locating humans or animals caught under wreckage).

Ongoing Support – Ongoing support involves fostering a sense of community in those who have made it through; developing a plan of ongoing shamanic intervention for all beings affected in the disaster; conducting regular group and ceremonial work; and befriending displaced spirits of the damaged land through the transition period by singing, making offerings, prayers, simple rituals, and offering friendship and a listening ear.

Spiritual Recovery and Maintenance, Seeding the Site – Seeding the site includes the work of planting seeds, with real viability for bloom, in which the ongoing spiritual tending can be assumed by those living in that area. This can be a long process with various times when people are benefited by charging the spiritual fires and dipping into the network of non-ordinary helpers; it's relating time to the very natural process within us. Some healing needs time to emerge on its own. We can't do everything in the first days or weeks after disaster strikes.

Anniversary – It is important to commemorate the disaster for those who lived through it or lost loved ones. This involves affirming the re-ordering/healing that has occurred while acknowledging and blessing the forever-changed, and making a commitment to return to the site (in journeys and ceremonies) later, maybe a year later, to tend the growth. The long aftermath of disasters is something shamanic practitioners should be addressing.

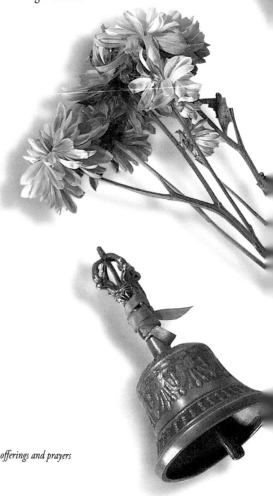

Sound, scent, and light can be useful tools when giving ritual offerings and prayers to damaged land. Photo by R. Short © 2010.

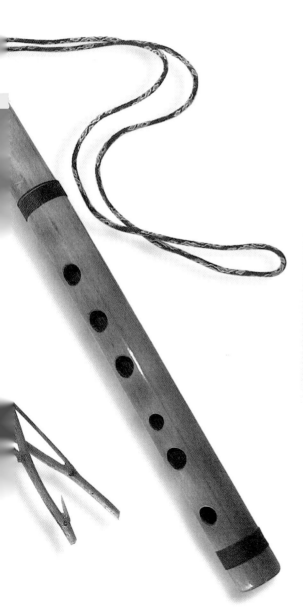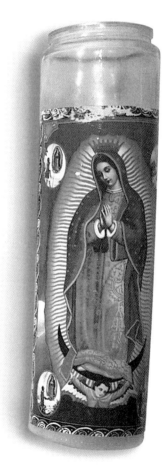

Ethical Considerations
Tom Cowan, PhD

Before embarking on any Shamanism Without Borders activities, we believe that practitioners should ponder the questions below and come to some resolution for themselves so that the work comes from a place of personal integrity.

— What ethical considerations apply and do not apply in the midst of death, chaos, and confusion?

— What Beings need to give their consent before we can work with them or their land?

— If we were physically present at a disaster in a land with a strong shamanic tradition, could we find ways to cooperate with local shamans, assuming they were not killed or injured?

— How do we work in areas that may never have had a strong tradition of shamanism or no longer have one?

— What kinds of shamanic tending can we do remotely?

— What ethical guidelines apply or do not apply when working remotely at a time of crisis?

— Are there ways to provide shamanic assistance to people of a different culture than our own with their own understandings of life, death, spirits, and wellbeing?

— What kinds of shamanic activities could be helpful during the disaster, after the disaster, during the recovery, and to mark the anniversaries of these events?

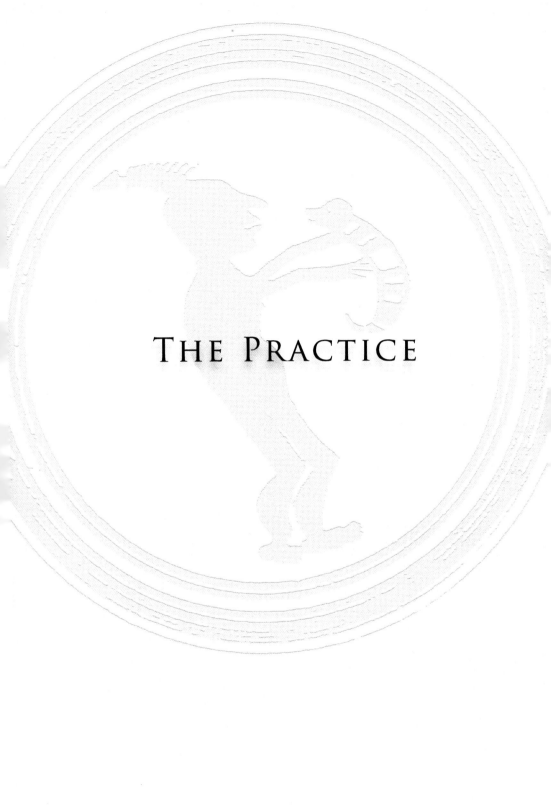

The Practice

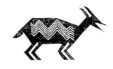

Working with Shelter Animals

Carol Proudfoot-Edgar, CSC

In the fall of 2008, I offered a weekend workshop at the Los Angeles East Valley Animal Shelter, the purpose of which was to see how our shamanic healing practices might be applied to animals left in shelters. Since we had limited time, we chose to focus on the canine population. However, with some variation, what we did could be applied to any other animal population within a shelter. A complete description of this weekend, along with responses from Circle participants can be found at the web pages titled Kindred Companions at my website: www.shamanicvisions.com. Based on this work, I offer the following guidelines for anyone interested in pursuing this particular way of practicing Shamanism Without Borders.

Preparation

Identify shamanic practitioners in your community who would be interested in this type of shamanic outreach. Send them a note regarding a time and place where you can gather for preparatory work.

Once gathered, journey regarding your focus (animal work) and see what helping spirits will assist you. Learn if there is some specific thing that the individuals and/or the circle should do in preparation for going to the shelter. Find out what totemic object to take with you and/or if you should take any type of crystal or stone. This is also a time to have conversations about the nature of this work and specific attitudes towards shelters.

It is important to understand the group is going to the shelter, not with the purposes of adopting animals, but to assist animals already there — such assistance could well result in the animal eventually being more adoptable. That is, by healing some of the wounds animals might feel (fear of humans, sense of betrayal), the animals might become more approachable when others who are seeking to adopt an animal visit the shelter.

Separate any political agenda one might hold from doing the shamanic healing work. For example, some of us are opposed to euthanasia. I am not arguing against this position but simply indicating that this is a different agenda. More doors will open to this work if we come with clarity that we are there to do healing work with the animals. We can participate with this clarity if we have had an opportunity to share our concerns and then put aside those not directly involved with the healing work.

Connecting with Shelter Staff

Someone in the circle needs to visit the animal shelter(s) in your area to get permission to do this healing work. Some shelters may be reluctant while others are eager for this support. In the initial encounter, it is useful to have a write-up describing what your group is planning to do at the shelter.

Often the hierarchy at these places means you meet with one person and they need to take the proposal to their immediate employer. It can take anywhere from one to four months before the shelter supervisor responds. In the meantime, it can be useful for members of the group to visit the shelter. There is a large turnover of animals in most shelters but the rhythm of the day and the structure of the shelter remains the same. Knowing this rhythm and the layout may be of invaluable assistance because your presence and healing activities can be aligned with the pace of the day that the animals are now experiencing.

It is important to develop a good relationship with one or two of the shelter staff and this can be done when visiting there.

Working within the Shelter

If at all possible, it's wise to have some meeting space at the shelter available to you for the hours you are there. If this is not available, then find some place close to the shelter (or even outdoors by the shelter) where you can meet.

Before the circle gathers, ask folks to bring a chair, journal, drums and rattle, and some totemic object that represents or is imbued with the spirit of the animals.

The first step in this work, as with all shamanic healing activity, is to transform ourselves so we can be conduits for Spirit. This means doing the ceremonial work that grounds the circle with Spirit and with each other. This also means asking what helping spirits will guide you in your work with the animals. It is important that Spirit and our specific helping spirits are with us when we enter the areas where the animals are kept. The animals sense; they know; they welcome this invisible help and they know if you are one through whom spirits are working on their behalf.

Various healing activities can be done once we are with the animals and with the help of the shelter staff. As examples, some will be listed here based on my experiences. These are only suggestions. As we do this work, if we share with one another, we will increase our range of known possibilities — all to the benefit of the animals. So I encourage posting any work that you do and informing the SSP shamanic community of what you have discovered and learned.

Examples of Healing Work in the Shelter

Signature Sound

Develop a "sound signature" of your presence; animals quickly bind sounds to behavior. This is a survival mechanism. I have found that a light sounding rattle is so useful as can be a specific song hummed while moving among the animal enclosures. If you rattle as you enter, rattle when first approaching some animal, and rattle while working with an animal, they will quickly come to associate the sound of the rattle with "good things happen" and/or "love appearing to me." After one afternoon of doing this, we discovered that the next morning when approaching with our rattles, the loud barking one hears from desperate animals completely disappeared and there was the silent expectations of "love appearing" that settled over the shelter. This is one reason why we must be judicious in our use of our rattle so that it is not used all the time but when we are specifically attuned to their needs and walking in our healing modality.

No Expectation Posture

Sitting beside the locked gate enclosing the animal, with no expectation that they behave in any particular way, establishes a reassuring relationship with an animal. Too often abuse of these animals is done in ways in which they simply don't understand what they have done wrong. This can develop an attitude of fear towards humans and not knowing how to behave. If we can sit beside their cage with love exuding from our beings, this allows them time to decide how they want to respond and to come from the center of their own being. Some animals may want to be petted and spoken to. Others may hang back from any contact and watch you with fearful eyes. Whatever your first response, it's important to simply convey, "I am here for you."

Responding with Specific Shamanic Help

The first round of going through the shelter should involve seeing as many different animals as appropriate to the circle's timing. Until we have done this, we may never be sure about what animal there that day is waiting for us. We know from synchronicity that once this process is set in motion, there will probably be some animal that seems to just be waiting for us or for a specific person. We won't know this if we stop with the first animal we see.

However, remember these are just suggestions and the first animal we encounter may be exactly the one we are to spend the entire time with!

Most of the processes involved in human-to-human shamanic healing are the same when applied to animals. For example, using some method for "seeing" (scanning) the animal for places of wounding, for soul loss, or loss of power. They are no different from us in terms of the range of hurt. The primary difference is that we don't speak their language and they do not speak ours although they can interpret from the tone of our voices. As with humans, they respond profoundly to touch.

Working with animals means applying a combination of direct and indirect healing (some might call the latter long distance or remote healing). From this perspective, objects such as crystals can be useful in holding, receiving or in sending during the healing.

Another difference in terms of actual wounding is that more animals are going to experience loss of home than are humans. From my experience, animals can sometimes give you pictures of their neighborhoods (from which they strayed) or some indication of where they belong. Often they seem to be waiting for their human guardians to appear and take them home. We can help with this wounding by conveying in our healing that "every human is home to you" or finding and returning their souls.

In some shelters, it is possible for a circle to work directly with the animals using the animal exercise areas. Being able to do hands on healing is preferable just at it is with humans. This is why establishing a good relationship with the shelter staff can be so important. If they understand and welcome your interventions, they often will do everything they can to ensure your ability to work directly with specific animals.

Walking Prayers among the Shelter Animals

In our first circle session, we discussed the power of prayer and what it meant to be a Walking Prayer as we moved through the shelter. Participants journeyed to see if there was some specific prayer that Spirit wished them to be making as they walked. This is analogous to a blessing of the animals and the deep understanding that whatever is blessed is amplified; the "Blessing Way" is held in such profound respect by shamanic peoples because it is based on the belief that blessing some being amplifies the health of that being and acknowledges that each being has a home on this planet Earth. At the end of our weekend, various participants commented on how powerful it was for them to experience themselves as Walking Prayers and their perception that the animals responded to them with increasing receptivity and trust.

I recommend that individuals and groups doing Shamanism Without Borders work discover how to hold themselves and walk in prayer. When we thus walk, others within our ambience feel the touch of love appearing and being made known. For many that experience of love is the initiating moment of learning how to move with less fear, less distrust, and confidence that there is a place for them here and now.

It is also important to make prayers for the staff of the shelter and just before departing after the healing work is done, bring the staff together – sing to and for them – perhaps rattle them and supplicate Spirit to care for and bless them in their shelter work. In this way, we are also tending our care to the ongoing caregivers. Whatever we can do in this regard is of benefit to the entire shelter.

Following Through

Two main issues can arise for individuals doing this kind of shamanic work in an animal shelter. Not surprisingly, we come to be connected to the animals we have met and especially with those for whom we have done some healing. Equally important, the animals become connected to us. How does one honor this new relationship? Again, one can draw parallels with shamanic healing between humans. If at all possible, it is most satisfying to be able to return to the shelter either as a group or as an individual. There may still be some animals at the shelter with whom you worked in your circle.

It is helpful to remember your signature sound (e.g. rattling). If some of these animals are still there, they will inform the new arrivals that this sound is positive. Some of us found that we wanted to make shelter visits in our local area part of our ongoing shamanic practice. Two women in the group returned to their community and have set up their own weekend of healing with their local shelter.

Create web pages where you can share among yourselves and others what you are discovering in this work.

We practice shamanic healing because we care about relieving suffering – we care about bringing compassion and peace into the world. And this means we seek to move with an open heart. Such openness can lead to real wrenching of our emotions when we encounter animals that have suffered because of what humans have done to or with them. Their fear of us can be heartbreaking for the eyes that look in fear tell us "you brought me suffering." The desperate yearning to be taken home by you can indicate how starved they are for a sense of place and that you can provide this for them. Whether they are at the shelter because they have been abused or because their previous owners cannot keep them, each one has a way of striking our very beings with a sense of responsibility — that is, with a sense that we should respond and be responsible for them.

This can lead to some individuals believing they must adopt a particular animal at the shelter. Some of us would like to take every animal home with us! But that's not really the purpose of doing shamanic healing work in the shelter. I strongly recommend that if such inclinations arise, the individuals be encouraged to wait — to give some time for reflection, journeys, and assessment of one's situation to make sure this is the action to take. It's important to remember that these animals have already lost one home, and the best outcome for them is to find a good home that has as much permanence as possible.

Again, this is where the human and animal parallels are so fascinating: we can go to an orphanage to work with the children, but this doesn't imply that we commit ourselves to adopting one or more children.

The issue of our limitations, of our humility in the face of much suffering, is one that usually surfaces in this healing work. Being able to share, to journey about and yet stay strong in our work are processes that can flourish when people work together. Doing this work alone can be very depleting. That's why I encourage people doing any type of Shamanism Without Borders to practice with a circle or at least one other person.

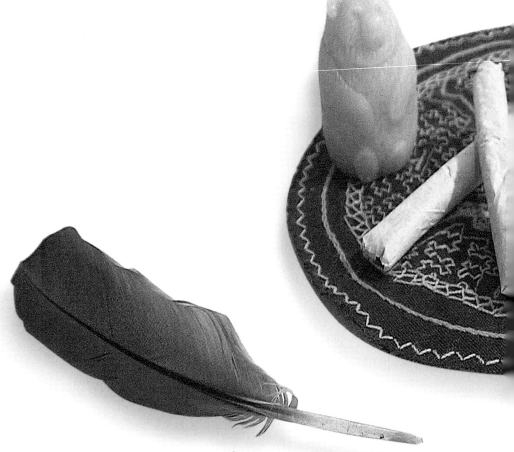

I have a vision that in each city or community where a shamanic circle exists, some time during the year is given to healing work in one's local animal shelter. It could even be combined with St. Francis' Day of Blessing the Animals. This is now a major day throughout the US in terms of our collective consciousness; the animals need our blessing and to the extent that we bless, so are we blessed.

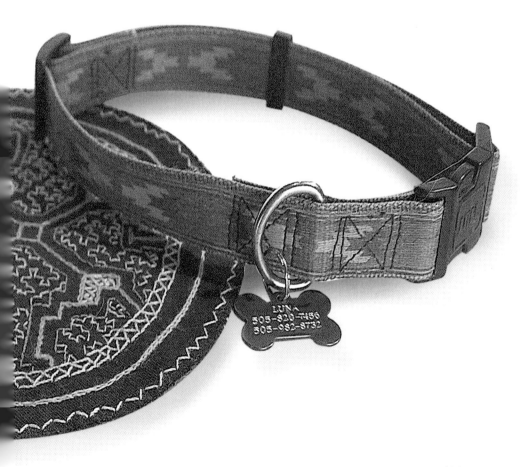

Totemic objects and shamanic tools can be useful in preparation for work with animals and to help establish a ceremonial space. Photo by R. Short © 2010.

Healing at the Scene of an Accident

José Stevens, PhD

In February 2010, I was leading a mixed group of twenty-seven people from six different countries on a memorable spiritual journey to the Lake Titicaca region in Southern Peru and Northern Bolivia. This region is notable to shamans around the world as being the new feminine spiritual center of the planet, recently transferred from the more masculine Tibet. After visiting transformational sites on the shores of Lake Titicaca in Peru, we crossed over into Bolivia by bus to visit Tiwanaku, a most powerful ceremonial site of a pre-Incan ancient civilization, but we arrived in heavy El Ninõ rain, too late in the day to have an adequate visit. Hastily we reworked the schedule with the bus company and agreed to overnight in La Paz and return the next day to Tiwanaku. Well rested, we returned to the site and offering coca leaves and tobacco, we respectfully asked permission from the spirits of that place to be there for a brief time.

We experienced an extraordinary morning exploring this ancient pilgrimage place still holding great power and teachings. We were fortunate to have an additional guide, provided by the site, who understood our orientation and who led us in a special ceremony to complete our experience there. Afterwards, we all gave each other heartfelt hugs and felt a deep connection to one another and the place itself. Tired and hungry we had a long lunch and just as we were leaving it started to rain. The plan called for us to retrace our steps to La Paz and then head on to Copacabana where we had reservations for the night at a good hotel.

My daughter Anna and I were sitting in the front of the bus and I noticed that the little jump seat in the very front next to the driver was empty so I called out that anyone wanting a good view could take turns sitting there. Tory, a Buddhist teacher from Colorado, volunteered and for some eerie reason I teased her saying, "First to the scene of the accident." She gave me a not-too-pleased look, with good reason as it turned out.

As the bus headed out to the highway, our spirits were high but soon most of the group began quietly processing their experience of the morning. The rain intensified and the bus began to navigate the steep terrain of the Bolivian highlands. We began to head down a steep hill with a long curve. With my elbow on the armrest, I was propping up my head on my hand, and closing my eyes, I began to doze off.

The next few moments are still somewhat confusing for me because although I had my eyes closed I somehow knew exactly what was taking place. A *collectivo*, a van packed with Bolivians, was passing a series of slower *collectivos* going uphill on the mountain curve we were heading down. By the time he spotted our bus heading toward him he did not have time to finish passing, so in his effort to get back in his lane, he crashed into the *collectivo* he was passing and sideswiping us, crashed into the driver's side of our bus. I remember hearing a tremendous sound of impact and before I could open my eyes the huge front windshield of the bus exploded and I felt like someone was tossing a bucket of popcorn onto my face and body. When I opened my eyes I was covered in sharp fragments of glass and the front windshield was completely shattered with shards of glass hanging like stalactites from around its rim. It was totally evident that safety glass was not used in Bolivian buses. The bus was still moving but very slowly now as the driver fought with the steering wheel to bring the vehicle to a halt before it slid into the deep rain gutter and turned over. I could see blood on his face but fortunately as it turned out he had only two minor cuts above his eye and on his chin.

I quickly looked to see what happened to Tory and saw her stand up shaking voluminous amounts of glass from her hair, face, and body. She had her eyes tightly closed and was concerned she had glass in her eyes. Glass shards had penetrated her seat all around where she had been sitting but none had penetrated her body. Again, it turned out she had no injuries other than two tiny punctures on the backs of her hands. I looked around to see about the other passengers. Everyone seemed to be in a state of shock, shaking the glass that had flown at eye level everywhere in the bus. One of our passengers received a slight cut to the bridge of her nose and was beginning to bleed. Other than that there were no cuts, broken bones or injuries to anyone in the bus. Although Anna and myself had received a high powered and massive shower of glass to our faces and bodies, neither of us had the slightest scratch on our bodies, even as we shook out all the glass that had gone down our necks under our clothes.

I staggered off the bus still shaking glass off me and miraculously the rain had almost stopped coming down. Cars were stopping and within minutes, mysteriously, two ambulances came out of nowhere and carried off two of the passengers of the *collectivos*. We were later to hear that there were no serious injuries and the passengers were mostly treated for shock. Most of our passengers disembarked and moved away from the bus to get the fresh air and freedom of the outdoors. Enrique, our Shipibo teacher and friend from the Amazon, produced a *mapacho* (jungle tobacco) and began smoking it to clear the *susto* (trauma). Soon everyone was blowing *mapacho* smoke on themselves and each other to clear the shock. This was the first time I had had the opportunity to use a *mapacho* so immediately after a trauma and was quite impressed at how well it worked.

As I wandered among our group I was amazed at how clear everyone was. Many were laughing and joking and commenting on the absolute miracle they had just experienced. A few got the shakes and became tearful as the shock was released in their systems. Everyone helped one another, no one freaked out, no one lost it and got hysterical, no one got angry, no one was injured badly and, most of all, no one died.

As we were waiting for another bus to arrive we had an hour or so to spare so a number of the group hiked up the embankment to say prayers and do personal work. I decided to walk up the road to clear the whole scene of the accident of *hoocha*, what the Q'ero people of the Andes call the low amplitude, inharmonious and heavy patterns being held there. The first thing I noticed was that there was construction going on by the side of the road and that the energy of that section of road was disrupted. After asking the local spirits about this they told me that this curve in the road marked a major *ceke* or ley line coming from Tiwanaku and going southward. This *ceke* had been cut by this relatively new road and thus was holding a pattern of disruption. Unfortunately the road had been constructed according to modern practices and none of the local land spirits had been consulted or asked permission before building it.

The *ceke* appeared to be both natural and enhanced by the people who founded Tiwanaku. Asking the spirits what needed to be done, they told me that just by observing the cut *ceke* and grasping what had transpired, I was beginning the process of re-establishing it. They told me that Spirit, directed by a focused mind with intention, could work wonders almost instantaneously. They seemed very happy for the tobacco and coca leaf offerings that were being made by the group.

They guided me by indicating that I should put my attention on Tiwanaku and then on the destination farther south where the *ceke* wanted to go, identifying the two most local points of a long *ceke* that extended well into northern Peru and ultimately off the coast. Although I didn't exactly know what that destination was, it appeared to be a set of ruins that was an outpost of Tiwanaku. I then did as they suggested, reaffirming the link in my mind and feeling the power of the places as they reconnected. Although the road would continue to cross the *ceke*, reconnecting the two points was critical to erasing the temporary bottleneck at that curve in the road. The *mapachos* had cleared the *hoocha* already.

The next day we went by boat to the Island of the Sun and hiked to the moon temple where we had the opportunity to do a *susto* clearing ceremony. *Susto* means a fright, shock, or trauma in Spanish. Although we had smoked our *mapachos* at the site of the accident, shock must be processed by the body first before it can be entirely released.

Therefore one must wait a good twenty-four hours to remove *susto*. This is also accepted protocol in the practice of EMDR, an eye movement desensitization technique used in western psychology. The *susto* ceremony had several parts and included the Mayan practice of shaking out the *susto* in a kind of skeleton dance and hitting the ground to clear it. Then Enrique sang a susto clearing *icaro* that he knew and Anna and I helped him in blowing *Agua Florida* on everyone's head to clear out what was left of the shock patterns. We gave thanks to Spirit for helping us and protecting us and we were done. After that everyone seemed fine.

Several teachings are revealed by these events. First, there is no need to dramatize or feel any pain in the process of clearing the *hoocha* away from a troubled site or from people. Secondly, the process needs to be guided by the local helping spirits because they know what the problem is and what needs to be done to handle it. Third, the act of restoring balance may be very simple, an act of attention accompanied by will. I have found that local spirits don't complicate things like we humans like to do. In fact the whole process of restoring resonance and balance can be quite joyous even though the circumstances might be grim.

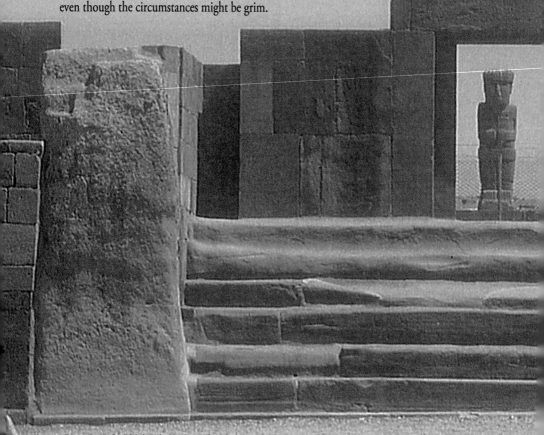

Tiwanaku, Isola del Sol, Lake Titicaca. Photo by Eugen Lehle © 2008 (GNU Free Documentation License). Photomontage by R. Short © 2010

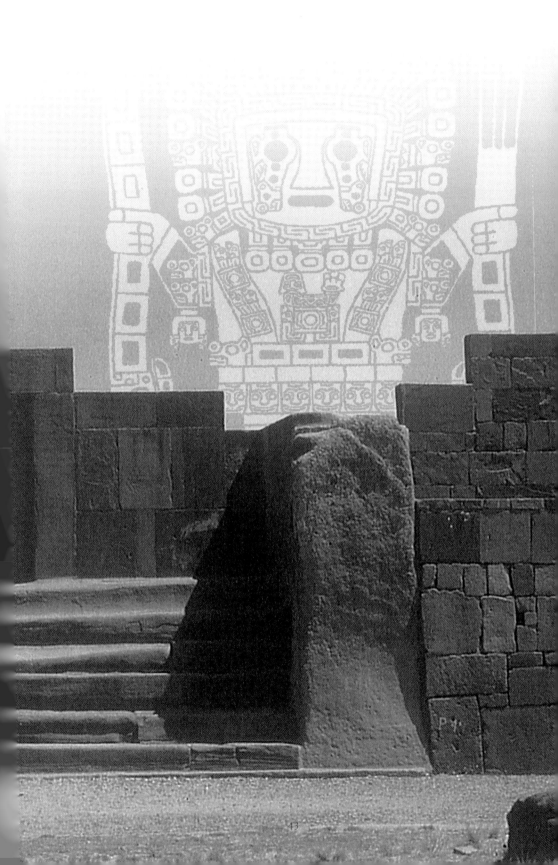

Healing When Multiple Accidents Occur in the Same Place

Pam Albee

In 2006, I was sponsoring a shamanic class to look at the ethics, layers, imprints, and occurrences of one particular intersection in our city. It had been in the paper as one of the state's worst/deadliest intersections. For our class project, we were going to spend the 12-hour class time learning about what had happened, what was continuing to happen, and how to perhaps help affect a healing in the intersection.

Our first journey was to ask our helping spirits the ethics of doing this type of work and who could give us permission to look at and get an overall view/diagnosis of what was happening in the intersection.

Then one by one, in separate journey's, we looked the various fields of landscape: elements and/or lack of, vortexes, *ceke* and ley lines, sacred sites, occurrences, imprints, power and/or soul loss, spirits, deceased souls, and/or entities stuck in the intersection in non-ordinary reality (NOR).

Each participant gave a detail accounting of his or her journey, which I wrote on a large chart. It was quite fascinating to see the chain of events — going back in time even before the road was there — to the present. It was easy to understand how drivers got distracted and confused while driving through the intersection because of the many NOR happenings that had occurred there.

The last journey was a healing journey for the intersection and NOR inhabitants, based on the information each participant received from their helping spirits. It was a blessed and emotional session for everyone concerned.

To my knowledge, that intersection has not been cited again as one of the worst/deadliest intersections in our state.

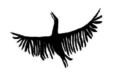

Finding Missing Persons
Pam Albee

THE FOLLOWING IS AN ACTUAL ACCOUNT of looking for a missing person using my helping spirits through shamanic journeywork. This event took place six years ago. Since that time, we have found three missing pets (gone for over a week) and worked with local search-and-rescue authorities to help locate missing bodies for cold homicide cases.

Years ago a colleague called me to do a journey for her friend whose husband had gone on a motorcycle ride at 8:00 am that Friday morning and not returned.

Friday 8:00 pm

It was 8:00 pm and there had been no word from Gary, which was out of character for him. Gary rode motorcycles for twenty years and was a good rider. The weather was turning and Gary had been taking a well-known 50-mile loop as his last ride before putting the bike away for winter. He was 67, in great health and retired. His wife of 45 years was panicked and had no idea what could have happened to him.

Friday 8:25 pm

My journey intention was "to find Gary and his motorcycle." I was familiar with 12 miles of the area he rode. My helping spirits took me to a field, where I could see an impression of where Gary had walked across the field and into a large group of deciduous trees. I was taken to a small wood brown shack/shed. There I saw Gary slumped in a chair — his eyes were closed and an angelic form appeared to be doing a Healing Touch (an energy based modality similar to Reiki) technique on him. There did not appear to be any injuries or blood, so I was not sure whether he was alive or deceased. The angelic helping spirit continued its work. Gary's face and hands were slightly grey in color and after a short while began to turn pink. I asked the helping spirit if he was alive, but got no response. I watched for a while trying to make sense out of the information. After the journey, I called my colleague. She was sad to hear I didn't have any concrete news for her and her friend. The authorities called off the search at dusk, much to everyone's distress.

Saturday 11:00 am

The next morning friends and family went out to physically search for Gary. The police sent rescue searchers and I went off on my own to look. When I was about 2 ½ miles from the accident scene (found on Sunday), I began to have severe chest pains. I kept asking Gary to show me where he was. The "loop" went through a small village and turned back towards town. Roughly one-half mile out of town, the chest pain went away. So I turned around and the chest pains returned. For two hours I searched the area back and forth driving five miles-an-hour looking over the edge of the road. I began to get a little frightened of the chest pains, wondering if they were mine or signs from Gary. After four hours of searching, I was exhausted and returned home – with no chest pain.

Saturday 7:00 pm

I journeyed again and saw the same exact scenes I had in my previous journey — Gary walking across a brown, dry, grassy field into deciduous trees along a creek and into the old brown wood shack/shed where the angelic helping spirit was still doing Healing Touch on him. Although his coloring looked normal, his eyes remained closed. Again I had no indication of whether he was alive or not. The helping spirit did not answer my questions. There was no word from the other searchers and again the search was called off at dusk. The State Patrol planned to have "air support" search for Gary on Sunday.

Sunday 10:00 am

I met a friend at my office who also journeys and asked if she would journey on Gary's behalf with me. I stopped short of telling her anything about my journey to see what she might get. We both journeyed and I again saw the same things I saw in my first two journeys. However, this time Gary was sitting on a log near the trees. He stood up when he saw me and smiled. He looked very peaceful, turned and walked into the trees and disappeared. I got quite emotional, feeling I perhaps had just witnessed his passing. My friend reported seeing a "man walking across a field into some trees" and saw a creek in the woods with a brown shed. She also saw a culvert with water and light colored pavement. I then told her of my three journeys, my search the day before and the chest pains I experienced.

Sunday 12:30 pm

My colleague called to let me know the authorities had just found Gary's body. I asked for the exact location. We drove along the same roadway I had taken the day before while searching for Gary. We came to the same spot where I experienced chest pains and

I showed her where I went back and forth looking for him as the pain came and went. Apparently (I couldn't see it the day before) there was a small side road which snaked backwards to another road which led to where Gary went off the road, approximately one-half mile from the small village. As we drove down the road, a tow truck passed us coming from the accident scene with Gary's damaged motorcycle on the back.

Sunday 1:45 pm

We arrived at the accident scene and both got goose bumps as we looked over the area and saw the brown grassy field and deciduous trees from our journeys. It was exactly as we had experienced it. I pointed to where I saw Gary walk into the trees. We walked the area looking for tire tracks and skid marks, looking for any kind of evidence that could help us understand what had happened. My friend noticed that right in that particular area the pavement was light colored, just as she saw in her journey. Intrigued, we then looked for the brown shack/shed we both saw in our journeys. Roughly one-half mile away along the paved roadway, hidden in the deciduous trees, was a small shack/shed. There was a creek near the shed and the culvert was just down the road. We sat and cried for a while – for the passing of Gary, gratitude for the loving care the angelic helping spirit was administering to him, the mystery of shamanic journeywork, and the awesome information our helping spirits were able to show us in search of Gary.

The Star Gazer Shamanic Moon Bear Project: Brave Compassion

Lora Jansson

"At the beginning of our first year, 39 bears were rescued. At year's end, twelve survived and thrived. Nine of the twelve had received shamanic work. No conclusions could be drawn, but the results were such that the Animals Asia Foundation (AAF) believed that the work had contributed to the health of the bears, and asked that we continue."

Passion is the fuel that feeds a shamanic project. My passion is for my helping spirit Bear. In my practice I do regular journeys asking my helping spirits how I can best honor them. Bear's request one day was "help." So I set upon a long journey through ordinary reality, one guided by intention and love, and driven by ethics. The result is The Star Gazer Shamanic Moon Bear Project. The Star Gazer Shamanic Moon Bear Project (SGMBP) is now entering its third year of service to Asian Moon Bears rescued by the AAF from lives of torture at "bear farms."

At these farms, captured bears, sometime quite young, are imprisoned in solitary, coffin-sized cages, and sometimes iron girdles. The bears are violated by a catheter inserted into the gall bladder under unsafe and unsanitary conditions; this process is done while the bears are conscious, and no anesthesia is administered. Trapped, with legs often sticking through cage bars, the bears are under-fed and under-watered. They are often kept for years in darkened barns and basements; line after line of the cages hold bears, and their bile is milked from the bears regularly.

Vets that attend rescued bears in the AAF Rescue Centers in China and Vietnam are amazed at the miraculous strength of these bears to have even survived their abuse for weeks, let alone years or decades.

Why do these violations take place? The bear bile, produced from the gall bladder, has been used as a medicinal agent in Chinese medicine for centuries, and is also sold on the black market. In the past twelve years, the AAF has made great progress in changing the social, political, and legal issues concerning these bears. No new bear farms can be established in China now. Still, 7,000 Moon Bears live throughout Asia in brutal captivity.

The SGMBP serves the AAF Moon Bears through actively seeking shamanic cures to restore power to these bears. In this paper, I will talk about the impetus to start the project, the mechanics of the project, and the ethics of doing this work.

Ethics and Intention

Ethical considerations must come first in any shamanic project that seeks to serve. Ethics and intention precede action, and actions and process can grow organically if ethics and intention are clarified and unified.

Each bear must give his or her implicit permission before shamanic work can begin. No being should ever receive shamanic work before permission is given. That rule, in my ethos, applies equally to all sentient and nonsentient beings. I would not work for a person or a tree without permission; permission is mandatory, and especially important for these bears who have suffered because people treat them as commodities. It is rational to expect that a rescued Moon Bear might reject a service offered by a human, and it is important for every worker to acknowledge that every bear has every right to do so. I think it of note to mention that while journeyers must often take several journeys to receive permission, no bear has ever refused shamanic work.

The intention of the project is to provide shamanic cures through the helping spirits to tortured Asian Moon Bears rescued by the AAF. Only shamanism is used in the project. While other spiritual practices may be very worthy, workers cannot mix other spiritual healing modalities with shamanism when they work with the bears. When they have tried, the work goes askew, and the integrity of the relationship with the bears is muddled. In three years, most of the times when the work has slowed or become strained is when practitioners try to marry shamanism with other practices.

I have not journeyed on why combining practices is not effective; it is an observation after watching a total of 51 workers interact with over 75 bears , and seeing when work starts to become muddled or confused either in outcome or by admission of the bear worker.

My position is that when you work with the helping spirits guiding your every action, you are using a very elegant, streamlined, and time-tested methodology. Introducing another modality mixes methodologies in such a way that the person doing the work has to become the ersatz captain of the ship. It is obvious to me that when you are working with shamanism, the helping spirits must remain in charge.

Each bear has her/his own dedicated worker. These bears have been tortured by humans, and are extremely sensitive. At the beginning, it was logical to assume that it would take time and extreme gentleness on the part of the journeyer and her helping spirits if a bear was to give permission to receive shamanic work. Often in this work, merging with a helping spirit or adopting a form other than human is the only way a bear will accept a worker. It is fascinating to see the many ways the helping spirits have to approach the bears to solicit their permission.

Later in the process, once the work is steady and the bear and worker have a solid relationship, it is between the worker, the bear, and the helping spirits to determine when – and if – the services of a drumming circle can be productively introduced. This creates a direct accountability, which is necessary in the work.

For many reasons relating to the way the AAF operates as well as the critical condition of the bears, workers agree to work with a bear for one year when they sign up for the project. At the project's inception, I had noted while studying the flow and work of the AAF that they routinely rescue a group of bears in January/February of every year. It can take a long time for a bear to be well enough to graduate from pen to den, if the bear can be saved at all; often, many months pass before a bear has healed enough to enjoy and to be functional within the boundaries of the AAF Rescue Centers.

This is a shamanic project ministered with love and compassion for the greatest good of all. It is not a study. This project exists solely to serve the injured Moon Bears through the power of shamanism. Validation of the efficacy of shamanic work, quantifiable information as might be gained by gathering statistical data, are not of interest to this project.

Certainly affirmations from the AAF, expressions of gratitude, encouragements to continue the work are all wonderful strokes for us to receive, but for on-going information about each bear's status, there is a blog on the AAF website we all read to stay abreast of the latest news; the bears' progress is our project feedback. Once or twice a year the AAF sends us specific project reports, which are always gratefully received by all of us.

At the end of the first year of the project, when there were no new avenues to explore to find volunteers to work on the project for another year, I implored Bear to find a way to continue the work if the work pleased Bear. That week, Susan Mokelke, executive director of the Foundation for Shamanic Studies (FSS), offered to run information about the project in the FSS Journal. It is only because of this support that potential shamanic volunteers found out about the project. This happy debt to the FSS can never be repaid.

Project Paradigm and Structure

In 2008 I had been following the work of the AAF for eight years when I decided to write them a letter asking if I could initiate a project that would enable the rescued Asian Moon Bears to receive shamanic cures. I described shamanism, and included a paper I wrote, which is used by many practitioners and teachers to introduce prospective students and clients to our modality; the article is called *A Practical Guide to Shamanism*.

The intention was to acquaint the AAF with basic shamanic precepts and practices, illustrating how shamanic work might be curative for recovering bears.

Some months later they wrote back inviting me to start such a project. I began to e-mail all of my shamanic peers in my FSS Three-Year Training Program and other Three-Year classes asking them to please forward my requests for volunteers. I will always be especially grateful to those first people who saw merit in the work, and who worked on the bears' behalf to spread the word.

Thirteen brave souls volunteered that first year to work for a group of newly rescued bears at the AAF Rescue centre in Chengdu Centre, China. None of us knew what to expect when we started the journeys. We could never have anticipated the intensity of the work, and the remarkable changes that we all went through as a result of the work.

It is important to note that communications from China to us about the bears were, and are, few. It was in that first year that most shamanic workers discovered unease about working for long periods of time without approval or feedback, apart from that given by the helping spirits.

When I journeyed on this, the spirits told me this: feedback is not important. The work is important. The bears' health would not be helped by feedback; it was only the practitioner who needed assurance. I was told that in other times, shamans would not expect to hear back from their clients. I was told not to treat this lack of continuous feedback as a problem. The helping spirits said it was important to only do the work as the helping spirits counseled.

This was a seminal teaching, and important to the focus and survival of the project in years to come. Because we are not trying to quantify information, run a double blind or any other kind of study, there is only one focus – to work with the helping spirits on behalf of the Moon Bears.

Can we claim that the cures the bears enjoy – whether that cure be death or health improvements — come only from shamanic work? No. Does that matter? No. What matters is that the bears receive the cures, and that they improve.

At the beginning of our first year, 39 bears were rescued. At year's end, twelve survived and thrived. Nine of the twelve had received shamanic work. No conclusions could be drawn, but the results were such that the AAF believed that the work had contributed to the health of the bears, and asked that we continue.

The second year 85% of bears that survived received shamanic work. In that year, the number of bears rescued – 13 – was smaller, and every bear had his or her own worker. This year, I do not have enough workers.

This and every year each bear workers write a report about every journey they take for a bear; the reports are narratives about each journey, and the journeyers' findings. Throughout the years, the number and kind of reports submitted for the project have changed. Currently bear workers submit weekly reports. The reports contain a synopsis as well as the full narrative of each journey taken that week; I compile the reports into one document and send them to the AAF.

I read every journey report that is sent to me. I then compile all the individual reports and send them to China. Each report is typically 25 pages.

This year we have 15 workers for a group of 19 Moon Bears rescued and brought to the Vietnam Rescue Center. In addition, seven "special need" bears, the matriarchs and patriarchs of the AAF, bears who have survived and thrived and who are now experiencing problems associated with aging, are also in need of workers. For this special group who live in China in a new house and yard devoted to them, I continue to solicit very seasoned and experienced shamans. So far, I have found one volunteer for this group.

Between the reading of the reports, answering individual questions, determining solutions to problems that workers encounter (which can range from the ordinary to the extraordinary), compilation and communications with AAF, the project takes a minimum of forty hours a month to properly administer.

Of course, my most frequent remedy for questions that I cannot answer is to journey. And it is the first suggestion that I always have for workers who are challenged or troubled by the work. Unerringly, this is the most efficient, transcendent, and swift way to answer any question.

Of course, this is not original or unique to this project, but it is the constant remedy to every problem encountered with the project. In fact, most problems develop because workers assume that they know how to diagnose or treat a problem without first journeying.

On Becoming a Bear Worker

When someone wishes to become a bear worker, he or she contacts me through my e-mail address – lorajansson@earthlink.net.

When I receive a request, I e-mail the Star Gazer Shamanic Moon Bear Guidelines. This eighteen-page document tells workers how to apply to the project, what will be expected of them, and some of the things we have learned throughout the three years of the project. Typically there is a flurry of questions before the worker starts with the first journey to get permission from a bear. Unique questions arise all the time. Sometimes, workers are stuck, and I will suggest a journey. Sometimes they just need to talk; they are often surprised by the depth and intensity of emotions they experience when they begin to work with their bear. This work teaches the absolute necessity of healthy shamanic boundaries.

It promotes what I call "brave compassion," which is the ability to hold great compassion for great suffering, to feel and really see the suffering, to do the work, but to leave the work in the shamanic studio when it is concluded. I would say that the most successful workers are those who feel enormous empathy for the bears, who do the work, and then do their own personal work to understand the unique teachings of the project. If done well, this work dismembers and remembers you into a stronger, more compassionate person. Shamanic work — especially work that is a marathon and intense as is true with this project — requires excellent boundaries.

One aspect of the project that is unique is anonymity. Unless a worker personally knows another worker, there is no contact between participants. When I work with each of the individual reports that bear workers submit in any given week, only the worker's first name is included in the final report. This policy was instigated by request. Occasionally, always with permission, I will share a journey report with the whole group for instructional purposes.

I believe the bear workers are the heroes of this project. This is intense work, and the commitment required is enormous. Week after week, in shamanic studios in the USA, Germany, and Australia, core shamanic practitioners lay down their blankets, go to their helping spirits to seek cures for their bear friend. The devotion that is consistently exhibited by these workers is inspiring.

Volunteer numbers vary from year to year. Last year I had so many volunteers, some of them never had the opportunity to work with a bear. This year I do not have enough workers; bears are waiting for help, and I just received word that ten more bears are being rescued right now, and will arrive at the China Rescue Centre at any moment. All of these bears need help now. If you are interested in becoming a bear worker, please contact me.

In Conclusion

Both Bear and the bears have gifted so many revelatory teachings to the shamanic workers and to me; most bear workers have told me that this is life-changing work.

In essence, this paper could be summed up this way: journey, journey, journey. Work with impeccable ethics. You need no guidance, permission, or instructions except from your helping spirits to begin a project like this one. Remember, you can journey on anything and everything.

When you are stuck, ask the spirits a question, and act on the answer. Be passionate and continually refine your intentions. Write an organization with whom you would like to partner. Write guidelines and solicit other journeyers who are inspired by the cause.

Work hard and unceasingly to serve. Love, respect, and serve the shamanic practitioners that volunteer. Create specific guidelines so that both those doing the work and those receiving it are served by it. Be prepared to understand that no matter how much you do (unless you can devote all of your time to your project), you may always be behind, and that that is reality. I do my best with this work when I remember those aspects of my job that are time driven — communications, reports, logistics — are important, but it is the ongoing work between worker and bear that is the soul of the project.

What is the most vital impetus for any shamanic project? Passion. Passion is what this work is really about. Bear is my beloved, and, for me, this project is a love story. I could never repay or thank Bear enough for all he has given me, my clients, and my students.

I started this project because Bear said a simple word to me in a journey — "help." Ironically, in the end, I do not believe that this project has given Bear or the Moon Bears nearly as much as he has given me since the project began. Perhaps that is because you blossom when you are with your beloved. You bring out the very best in each other. You grow in ways that you never could have anticipated when you are in a love affair.

The time, the sorrow, the exhilaration, the feeling that you are always behind, the joy – all make you better equipped to dive deeper, to do your best. It completely rearranges the notions of what it is to do shamanic work in contemporary society. Shamanic work should never have borders. To do this kind of work is not to practice shamanism, but to live shamanically. It is to embody the work in the world.

We have never been in greater need of passion. I hope this project demonstrates that there is not a cause out there which cannot be aided by shamanic work. Just like you, I am a core shamanic practitioner; if I can start a project like this, so can you. I believe that somewhere in the heart of all shamanic workers there is a passion that, if acted upon, could lighten the very nature of reality. That is something that cannot be constrained to borders. It is something that is wild and free that the soul and the spirits celebrate.

Please contact Lora Jansson at lorajansson@earthlink.net if you are interested in volunteering or learning more; more shamanic workers are needed.

Contact Animals Asia Foundation at www.animalasia.org to donate or find out more about their work. It is more extensive than I have been able to describe here.

Contact the Foundation for Shamanic Studies at www.shamanism.org for more information about their work.

I was honored that the SSP requested this paper from me about the Moon Bear project, and am very grateful for their interest. Having acknowledged their generosity, this paper is dedicated to Susan Mokelke and the Foundation for Shamanic Studies. As I have written, without the Foundation's assistance, and their willingness to publish on-going articles in the FSS journals, this project would have failed long ago. I am very pleased to finally be able to formally acknowledge their help, encouragement, and support.

Opposite: Moon Bear *by Don Hazeltine © 2010.*

LAND TENDING AT A WINDMILL SITE
Cecile A. Carson, M.D

SHAMANISM WITHOUT BORDERS, a project of the Society for Shamanic Practitioners (SSP), is based on the tenets of being in service through "shamanic tending" of areas that have been transformed through natural or man-made earth-events— and, in doing so, of not making assumptions of what is good/bad, right/wrong, shamanic/not-shamanic.

In June 2010, a small group of shamanic practitioners drove to a beautiful hilly area just outside Naples, NY, and parked in the sheltered driveway of the area's electrical substation. Farmland and homesteads were around with about 8 windmills in close proximity lining one of the ridge tops, with several dozen more on adjacent ridge tops. The buzz of the electrical substation was the prevalent noise, with an occasional car going by on the highway. We experienced the windmills as having a certain beauty as they stood waiting for wind -- alien, but also graceful. Our purpose was to make contact with the spirits of that land impacted by the construction and ongoing presence of the windmills to ask if and how we might be of service. We knew that shamanism asks us to work toward balance and right relationship among all parts of the great web of life, and that is what we focused on.

What follows is a composite report from our individual experiences with the spirits there, the spirits' response to us, and how we attempted to be of help.

SPIRITS OF THE LAND

There were several types of spirits that presented themselves. Guardian Spirits were there in a formless presence that felt welcoming. Two people experienced the Spirit of the Land as a very old and masculine energy that was immense, annoyed and forthright: "a giant of stone, earth, and moss, none too pleased to start with, who swung at me with its big rocky appendages." Another person was taken below ground to meet an ancient, healing circle of Beings working on a ritual of rebalancing.

Spirits' Messages

We discovered a great deal of concordance in the messages people received. The spirits said the construction work that was done had stopped much of the energy there from flowing, and the power spots that the earth blood flowed from had been clogged. If the windmills couldn't be removed, the spirits felt the ley lines and power places needed to be cleared so the Earth energy could flow once again.

The strongest concern expressed by the land spirits was about the harmonic vibrations caused by the windmills themselves during their operation. The vibrational energy of the land is ancient and slow—the bedrock is a particularly slow form of stone movement—but the windmills are high, tight energy. The place where the windmills are anchored to the ground is a zone of conflict between the two energies. The contradiction in vibrations was setting up a dichotomy that could prove to be a source of the bedrock giving way underneath. The water that permeates the region, seeping into the bedrock, could add to the dissonance and result in rock slide.

There were also multiple messages about the need for humans to learn to ask permission of the land before doing something like this, to work with the land on how the effect of our construction on the earth can be minimized, and to observe the proper rituals after construction to assure that what damage is done is healed. The spirits understood that humans build windmills as an alternative to other energies that could do more harm to the Earth, and they were willing to work with us but were clear they needed to be involved in the process.

For one member there was also a strong message from the spirits of the substation area where we parked that "the windmills are the least of our problems; it is the electrical substation that is doing great harm." They said electricity isn't "bad," and that we could journey to the Spirit of Electricity to ask how we can make better use of the power to mitigate the damage from the production of power. They also said, "Electricity has been in existence since the beginning of time; everything on this planet has oil and nuclear energy as well. It is what humans do with these elements that creates negative consequences."

The Tending

Several of us were guided to sing as a way of attending to the spirit of the hills there. The singing was profound and was a way to shift the energy of the land back into balance.

For another person, "My helping spirits began to work with the two kinds of energy of the land and the windmills, weaving them back and forth to create a sort of web or strand of the blended energies. Then with song and toning, we all lined up to send the new blended energy as a vibration down the corridor of the ridge top."

For two others: (1) "Where the wells of the earth blood, the places of power, were clogged, I was shown to reach down in, past the clog, to open the well. I could feel the Spirit of the Land walking with me along those lines. It rumbled a song as it walked. Afterward, others who had also been instructed to open those lines traveled down them singing, carrying the music in their hearts and opening the ways"; and (2) "I recall walking around the area and punching holes in the energy spots to release the energy that was building up; it seemed helpful."

One person lay down on the ground and felt the journey through her lower chakras. "I was taken to an ancient, visionary circle below the ground to witness their work, though not participate in it as they said that I had not yet achieved a state of balance able to handle the energy frequencies they were working with. They showed me how they were balancing the land at the base of the windmills so that the energies at the threshold were more in alignment with one another." They then invited her to return to learn their ways.

Aftercare

The spirits asked us to keep singing with them, to work with them again both in person and remotely. One person has gone remotely every week since the initial time, tending the land through singing. Although she found the energy there had skewed out of balance again, it was much less than initially encountered. The singing appeared to keep bringing it back into balance.

Part of aftercare is the impact of this experience on us as humans and co-walkers with all of life and what we will do with that experience. The Spirit of the Land's message to the group went in deeply: "Use the power generated from the windmills wisely. Do not waste, as my price for your progress is high."

In this work, there is also the potential to have a seemingly negative reaction to the Middle World work if we are not careful about being protected and attentive to our language and the framing of our questions. One person found herself having the experience of seeing her life force drain out of her temporarily to a nature spirit when she asked, "What can I do to help?" and introduced herself by name. "The spirit thought I was offering what I had that it needed -- my energy, my own special brand." Later the spirits gave her a message through another group member that she was demonstrating the same thing that they (the spirits) have experienced through the windmills' construction – a draining of the life force of the land.

Here is her reflection on the process after recovering: "Now, I know in my bodymind that the suffering of the Earth is at least partly due to our quest for more energy. How can I mindlessly return to taking the Earth's resources for granted? The answer to the question, 'What can I do to help?' is to stop squandering valuable resources and to make a decree: I will only take what I need from the Earth. I will return to the Earth respect, and the power of my intention to live my own divinity . . . This is a life's work."

Reflections from the 2010 SSP Conference

Tom Cowan, PhD, Bonnie Horrigan,
Carol Proudfoot-Edgar, and José Stevens, PhD

In June 2010, sixty shamanic practitioners came together for the Society for Shamanic Practitioner's (SSP) first foray into the Shamanism Without Borders (SWB) initiative. We gathered at Kennolyn Retreat Center near Santa Cruz, California. The intent was to explore how shamanic tending could heal the trauma caused by natural and/or man-made disasters that was still being held by the land or its inhabitants in the Santa Cruz area.

One way to think about SWB work is to compare it to holistic healing, which is founded on the principle that given the right conditions, the human body will always heal itself. Consider a broken bone. A physician will set the broken bone, lining it up and ensuring its stability, but it is the body, the bone itself, that actually knits itself back together. The physician has merely set up the conditions that allow the body to utilize its maximum healing capacities.

Given the right conditions, the earth and the animals and people who inhabit it will heal themselves. What we can do as shamanic practitioners is to remove the unseen barriers that prevent this self-healing. When we correct the flow of energy, perform a soul retrieval, awaken dormant spirits, usher wayward souls on their journey, forgive a transgression, soothe through song, or "see" what is there in its fullness, we are enabling self-healing. This is our work. This is the unique contribution that Shamanism Without Borders practitioners can make to the health of the world.

Choosing the Sites

To speak of "natural disasters" presents a challenge of definition and understanding. To speak of "healing" the land after a disaster also requires careful definition. In some sense natural disasters such as earthquakes and floods are perfectly natural events. We call them disasters because of the disruption they cause according to our human expectations. And in the long term the earth does not need healing; she will heal herself, although again, perhaps not in line with human expectations.

So we offer two concepts to help us understand what occurs in natural disasters and what we can or should do about them. First, we use the following as a working definition: A disaster is an event that creates a serious and sustained disruption of the normal life patterns of the land, waters, animals, and people. (We know of course that the word "normal" is subject to interpretation and to local conditions.) Second, we consider our response as shamanic "tending" which may or may not include regular shamanic healing practices as we might use them in other contexts.

Santa Cruz has had a long history of such disruptive events, which have come in the form of floods, earthquakes, mudslides, fires, and human violence. Prior to the conference, with these two concepts in mind, Carol Proudfoot-Edgar and Susan Gilliland carefully researched various sites in the area that displayed signs of continued deep distress and chose seven sites for the SWB teams to visit. Listed below are the sites with a brief history of why each was chosen.

Fire/Earthquake
Summit Fire and Nisene Marks Park — SWB Team Leader: Susan Gilliland

Major fires are a recurrent problem in Santa Cruz resulting in extensive loss of habitat for all affected. Although business properties are now more protected, the wildfires in the mountainous terrain of Santa Cruz County, especially in the last ten years, have resulted in extensive burning of vast tracts of wilderness. The largest wildfire-affected area in decades, the Summit Fire of 2008, was chosen as the site to tend: it destroyed 3,200 acres, including homes, and forced the evacuation of thousands of residents. Three years later, some people are still looking for their various companion animals (horses, dogs, cats, lamas) and the effects of this fire still burn in the psyche of the people living here.

Although minor earthquakes are frequent, the Loma Prieta Earthquake of October 17, 1989, was the most extensive in Northern California since the San Francisco April 1906 earthquake. The epicenter was located in Nisene Marks Park in Santa Cruz County. The quake killed seven people, destroyed much of downtown Santa Cruz, and residents throughout the county were faced with repairs to almost every single dwelling. Each year on this date, residents still gather to remember the Loma Prieta Earthquake and to remind themselves they live in an area where Earth "shakes herself" frequently. This group went to the actual faultline area located in Nisene Marks.

Polluted Rivers/Marine Sanctuary
20th St Beach/Lagoon and Moran Lagoon/Beach — SWB Team Leader: Sandra Hobson

Water, in its various forms, is a defining signature of Santa Cruz County. The health of the land and inhabitants is dependent on winter rains of 35–50 inches. Rivers coming from the mountains have carved deep canyons down to the ocean and in various areas, wetlands and lagoons have established themselves.

Years of periodic drought have led to more extended attention to careful tending of the reservoirs and marine sanctuaries in the area. After decades of ignoring the needs for protecting these special waterways that provide sanctuary for many species, Santa Cruz County has finally undertaken projects aimed at preserving them and improving the quality of these habitats. The water quality of these two beautiful lagoons and beach areas often dictates their closure as bacteria levels exceed safety standards. The pollution comes from the nearby sewage treatment plant, chemical-laden runoff water from the town, and the thoughtless dumping of trash by visitors to these areas. Working with lagoons is one way of connecting with the pollution of water all around this country, including the Gulf of Mexico.

Mudslides/Loss of Life
Love Creek Memorial Site — SWB Team Leader: Cecile Carson

The geology of Santa Cruz County includes extensive limestone, friable cliff sides, and hillsides vulnerable to mudslides. The very heavy rains upon which this area is dependent can, at times, produce devastating earth changes. This was the case in the 1982 floods, and subsequent Love Creek landslide, that occasioned international attention.

In this earth event, the entire top third of a mountain quickly released itself, moved down the slopes, and smothered entire homes and lives. This deadly combination of torrential rains and mud killed twenty people, including two small children whose bodies still remain beneath the tons of earth and trees. There is a memorial at this site that includes the children's toy box, and a request to "remember them." This site was chosen both to honor this request and to see what other tending might be needed there.

Troubled Past
Holy Cross Mission and Old Holy Cross Cemetery — SWB Team Leader: Lena Stevens

The first Santa Cruz mission, built on the banks of the San Lorenzo River, was flooded in 1791, driving the missionaries further up the hillside where they rebuilt. In 1840 an earthquake and tidal wave destroyed much of the mission. The cruelty of Father Andres Quintana and the revolt by the mission Indians (the Ohlone and Yakuts, who had previously lived freely along the river) are examples of a deep-running strain of violence and trauma that has occurred in and around the Mission.

The Old Holy Cross Cemetery is another example of this deep-running strain. In building the new mission (mid-1800's), it was determined that the graves at the new building site would need to be moved. Bodies of the Indians there were taken to what is now called Old Holy Cross Cemetery and put into one mass grave. The burial site itself was never given any marker or headstone to indicate whose remains are there. This unmarked site is surrounded by later graves well marked and periodically tended.

Santa Cruz County has endured a series of epidemics including the smallpox epidemic of 1868, the polio epidemic of the 1940s and 1950s, and the AIDS epidemic of the 1990s. However, the one that killed the most and left the most enduring memory was the flu epidemic of 1918. Known as the Spanish Influenza, this pandemic killed hundreds of people. The cemeteries have clusters of 1918 flu-death burials, in some instances including entire families.

Both the current Holy Cross Mission site and the Old Holy Cross Cemetery were chosen as places where ancestral spirits and the bones of previous generations of a place may wish to communicate to us and/or may need tending.

TROUBLED PRESENT
Beach Flats/Boardwalk — SWB Team Leader: José Stevens

The Beach Flats/Boardwalk is a nine-acre neighborhood site that represents the possible interrelationship between elements, boundaries, urban development, and serious problems of violence in our world today. This is an area of housing that is adjacent to the Santa Cruz Boardwalk which itself is at the ocean, on the beach. This area is well known for gang activity and multiple homicides each year. In the mid-eighties, this area came under the aegis of "affordable housing" requirements in Santa Cruz which eventuated in housing for low-income families and resulted in a mixture of diverse ethnic families with Hispanic and migrant farm workers as the primary residents.

The current proposed redevelopment of this parcel is the cause of major controversy between the locals and the City Council. It is home to 1200 residents who do not want to see their houses and community destroyed by the proposed redevelopment plans.

The group going to this site explored how the restiveness and violence in this neighborhood might be exacerbated by its very geographical locations. That is, adjacent to the Beach Flats neighborhood is the Santa Cruz boardwalk—a very popular site for both County residents and tourists, characterized by high traffic, noisy boardwalk rides, trashed grounds, and unending cacophony. The boardwalk itself is situated on the beachfront with the relentless crashing of surf against land and related beach activities. Given that the actual space is limited in each of these areas, how do the different activities that characterize neighborhood, boardwalk, and beachfront activity interface? And can interfacing be done in such a way as to bring more overall peace and balance to the Beach Flat inhabitants?

EPICENTER OF ALL DISASTERS
Downtown Santa Cruz — SWB Team Leader: Tom Cowan

Santa Cruz downtown has grown from a 1797 pueblo with a racetrack to a small downtown area characterized by its beautiful mall which houses both businesses and residents, thus making Downtown Santa Cruz a real community in the heart of the County.

The downtown area underwent extensive renovation and expansion following the opening of the University of California, Santa Cruz in 1964.

The area itself is a flood plain and until levees were built after the Great Flood of 1955, the town was frequently under water that poured over the banks of the San Lorenzo River situated now just above the town. After the extensive development of canals and levees, a river, once brimming with life, seems a pathetic being. How does one address the relationship between water and town and between river and land inhabitants? This is the major waterway that courses through the county, coming from the mountains, including Nicene Marks (epicenter of quake). Just as the earth quaking can destabilize an area, do these methods for controlling river's flow create an overall destabilizing effect?

Downtown Santa Cruz was the most severely impacted area from the 1989 earthquake. Three fourths of the town had to be rebuilt. One person died from collapse of a building. There is a large square hole at the top of the mall where a popular bookstore existed prior to the earthquake. Now, recently posted, is a large sign indicating that 50 luxury condominiums will be built on that space. Until a chain fence was erected two months ago, that hole-in-the-Earth was a site in which residents would gather for ceremony and construct murals. Periodically altars would appear reminding folks to "remember, remember.'"

Since its founding, the town has been characterized by a restive relationship between those who regard themselves as the "real or local residents" and those who are regarded as the out of towners or drifters. Given the benign weather climate of Santa Cruz, it has become a haven for the homeless and those simply wandering for multiplicity of reasons. The majority of the people seem to welcome both along with a desire to find peaceful ways of sharing the town and its resources. There are, however, the occasional altercations. Some residents bear signs that read, "Take back Santa Cruz" and engage in what they call " positive loitering." On May 1 of this year, violence erupted during a May Day celebration and 19 stores were damaged. The outbreak was blamed on anarchists and/or drifters.

The whole downtown area — both in construction and in daily living — has been shaped by major earth events and processes (e.g. water flow). What can river and quaking earth teach us about living together in Santa Cruz? Is there any way to ease and redefine the relationship between local and outsider that recognizes we share the same resources? Is there anything river needs from us?

Preserved Place of Power
Henry Cowell State Park — SWB Team Leader: Carol Proudfoot-Edgar

Places of power, the natural guardians of the earth and the headwaters of certain types of energy, are models for what health and wellness look and feel like. Every region has at least one Place of Power which functions as the keeper and provider of health for the whole area. Within such a place live the elders of the region. The elders themselves manifest the powers and health of that place, that ecological niche in the greater web.

The Henry Cowell Redwoods State Park is one such place. Looking much the same as it did 200 years ago when Zayante Indians once lived in the area, it is home to a centuries-old redwood grove and other old-growth woods such as Douglas Fir, madrone, oak, and ponderosa pines. The tallest tree in the park is about 285 feet tall, and about 16 feet wide. The oldest trees in the park are between 1400 to 1800 years old.

Given their lengthy lives, the redwoods here have seen and experienced more of what has occurred in this region than any other living being. And with their far-reaching, lofty stature, they can over-see beyond the edges of the place's boundary. Thus they can be forecasters of that which is approaching the place. Examining their annual rings of growth can provide details of how disease, weather, and human behavior impacted the health of the forest itself. Understanding how the beings in this park, and those in other places on the planet, carry wholeness can help shamanic healers as they reach out to sites in distress.

The Bones of the Gathering

Conference attendees were divided into seven smaller groups of approximately eight people each. Thursday night was spent together learning the history of the Santa Cruz area and the nature of the SWB work that was to come. A collective journey was taken to ask for the help of the spirits native to Santa Cruz as well as people's individual helping sprits.

On Friday morning the small teams met with their respective group leader to get acquainted with one another and engage in advance work that typically involved drumming, journeywork, and remote viewing to see what guidance spirit would offer. After lunch each team traveled to their assigned site to engage in prayers, rituals, and shamanic tending that would shift the energy and promote healing. This work lasted until evening. Friday night a prayer tree was erected and the group participated in a *despacho* ceremony. On Saturday the small groups gathered in the morning for further remote work for their sites. Saturday afternoon was filled with a spirit canoe healing for the BP oil spill in the Gulf of Mexico and in the evening, the group engaged in a Condolence Ceremony to release grief. After the smaller groups shared their site experiences with each other on Sunday morning, the conference ended with a snake dance.

The Bones of the Work

It is important to note that while the foundation for the work was the same for the seven groups engaged in the Shamanism Without Borders excursions, each group experienced something unique and each used different healing techniques to move the land, animals, and people involved in their respective site toward wholeness. It is also important to note that there was broad general agreement that having a community of shamanic practitioners working together created far more healing power than any one individual working alone could have generated.

Almost half the groups encountered a snake in their work, but never in a fearful way. Snake was welcomed as the carrier of the imprint and energy of transformation. Butterflies literally surrounded one group as they ended their healing work. Other animals that came to witness the healings were minnows, herons, ducks, seagulls, hawks, crows, squirrels, and rabbits.

The Love Creek team engaged in psychopomp work to usher the dead onto the next phase of their journey and release their imprints from the area so healing could occur for those still present on the earth. "The land itself at Love Creek was doing fine, but it welcomed us as 'walkers between the worlds' to come there to help heal and release the human energy of grief still hanging on in this place," one practitioner said.

The group working on the San Lorenzo River created a ceremony for restoring the proper flow of energy. They drummed and rattled softly. In turn, they each took three spiritual drinks from the "river" they had created on their altar. The first was for the river herself, the second for the downtown area, and the third for whatever else was needed. The entire group infused the river with the energy needed to fix disrupted lines that crossed the river at the bridge. They ended by toning, bringing light to the area, with special consideration for the area between the land and what has been built on top of it.

One member of this team received the following message from the river: "Rivers are created to be sheltering places and sources for life. From earliest times, people, animals, birds hover along our banks. They drink and refresh themselves. Wash the aches from their bodies. Relax. Today most people ignore or trash me. They can no longer drink from me. But the homeless still gather and live along my banks in ways similar to the earlier ages. In spite of their cluttered lives they are dear to me. They use me as a sheltering place much as I was created to be used. I am here to refresh them when they are hot and thirsty, cleanse them when they are dirty, soothe their fears when they are worried. I value them."

The group that went to the beach flats near the boardwalk discovered that elementals were playing an active role as spirit helpers. As one practitioner said, "The elementals strengthened our ability to listen from our core through our shamanic senses amid the distractions of the physical environment, to be open and flexible to what was possible with the resources at hand." This group felt a significant energy shift after a ritual was preformed.

The group assigned to Henry Cowell State Redwood Park went to specifically learn about places of power. They discovered that the trees have memories of how the region survived in times of disaster, information that could inform other plans for facilitating health. One member of the group chose to meditate instead of journey while in the park. When she returned from her meditation, she revealed her learning. "I was so surprised to find myself among a thousand redwood meditators." Then she smiled. "Now I know that it was no mistake that Buddha attained enlightenment beneath a tree." The group learned that one of the qualities of a place of power is duration of form.

On Saturday afternoon, the sixty SWB workers gathered together to summon forth a Spirit Canoe and travel to the Gulf of Mexico to render aid and healing. Upon the group's return, as the Canoe docked, the room felt hot and smelled of fumes. While transitioning from the Gulf to Santa Cruz, Wind Woman carried a message to Carol that we had, for that short time, extracted the toxic substances from the Gulf of Mexico and in so doing, had given some time and space — or breathing room — for healing for those present in that injured, perilous, and poisoned area.

Unlike some types of interventions, SWB healing work cannot be done in a single, focused session; the wounds we are dealing with are often nasty and vigorous, and they keep tearing the very fabric of life. Because of this very realization many of the SWB healing teams elected to continue working together through e-mail and skype.

Part of the healing work means developing patterns of living that honor the integrity of other living forms, and to walk with feet that leave healthy ground for those beings coming through hundreds and thousands of years from now. We may not be able to see those faraway descendants but each of us holds some knowing about what's needed for life-sustaining behavior. And our collective, shared response in using this knowledge is what it means to live in conscious shamanic community.

An Evolving Shamanic Community

As Carol Proudfoot-Edgar has pointed out, the days at the conference were characterized by a deepening awareness of the power of shamanic community. We are evolving together and our maturation as a shamanic community might actually be the very resource that enables us to respond to the troubles in our present age.

We live in a web of interrelations, and strands from any deep wound thread themselves throughout the world. Just like people wash off the oil that is coating birds, marine animals, and grasses in the Gulf, so too do these spiritual strands in the web need cleansing.

The Redwood Groves manifest community. The next generation grows beside the elders. Next to one of the ancient trees, a sapling, around 20 years old, is healthy; and beside it, a newly born is just emerging from the soil. The young are sheltered in their growing by their proximity to the trees surrounding them who have participated for 2,000 years in the creation of their forest community. We can use these "ways" to create and sustain our own community of those who practice shamanism.

The human community has been the primary recipient of our shamanic work for many years. Like an orphaned child, nature received the least direct attention and/or was the backdrop against which our activities occurred. For example, it was important to learn certain plant spirits because their medicine might be the source of healing for some individual.

Over the last fifteen years, however, we have slowly come to realize that our work must be grounded in doing whatever it takes to honor, heal, and preserve the community known as Earth and help sustain its diversity of beings and its very wildness.

The Shamanism Without Borders initiative calls us to turn our attention to conscious community-building: to see each and every being as having place. One of our challenges and opportunities is to have conversations and explorations about who we are and how we are as a shamanic community. We shall always be students but we are now called to be teachers, colleagues, and full time partners in the evolution of shamanism. This new perspective manifested at the gathering — we did not come together as students there to learn from a few select teachers. Yes, we had guides, but the group was clearly a gathering of fellow shamanic practitioners there to participate together in healing work. And that, in and of itself, was a powerful shift.

This is the evolutionary stage we have reached and it requires of us to continue building a community that is rooted in Spirit and within which individuals provide the necessary roles and functions as required by the collective.

To grasp how profoundly true this is means knowing that the "Age of the Individual" has passed. That paradigm may have worked for a different stage in our evolution but that era is gone. That doesn't mean there are not times when an individual may take center stage but we now know that the value and rights of the individual and the value and rights of the community of beings are inseparable.

As Carol Proudfoot-Edgar says, "We are neither powerless nor ignorant; we are not naïve or undeveloped. In collaboration with our helping spirits and the eternal compassionate powers, there is no trouble our shamanic community cannot help transform."

For more information about Shamanism Without Borders, please visit: www.shamansociety.org.

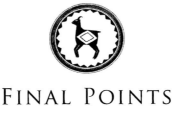

Final Points
Lena Stevens

Keep it simple

IN THE HEARTFELT DESIRE to be of service there can often be a tendency to overcomplicate. Elaborate rituals, unnecessary drama, and the need to fix every detail through an endless process can sometimes be the influence of the ego's need for self-importance rather than the result of clear listening and straightforward intuition. Always keep in mind the definition of responsibility as one of being able to respond. There is a fine line between responding to what a situation requires and inserting one's own mental process. Keep your motivation non-personal. The best way is to stay out of judgment about what you are guided to do. The minute you judge any of it to be good, bad, effective, non-effective, too simple, not enough, too much, you have made it personal. When in doubt, keep it simple.

The simplest and perhaps the most powerful way to begin anything is by saying hello. If you say hello to the land, location, spirits, ancestors, body of water or air space, you are creating a starting point for the work. In shamanic practice it is important to define your beginnings and your endings. Saying hello acknowledges the energies that exist, and sometimes just that in and of itself, is enough to bring about healing. Everything wants to be seen and acknowledged and the simplest way to do that is to say hello.

Once you have said "hello" and opened up the possibility for a deeper exchange, ask what, if anything, is needed. Then listen and hear with all your senses. Often you will find that something simple is what is being asked for, such as gratitude, a song, a prayer, an offering, or some other form of attention or communication. Don't overdo. Just do what is asked.

How do you know if work is needed?

If you say hello and are receptive without your ego or your own beliefs getting in the way you will know if there is something needed or not. Appearances can be deceiving and you may find that what appears to be ravaged and disrupted is actually in balance and performing a necessary service in the greater scheme and the larger picture. Never make assumptions. Natural disasters are often catalysts for change and happen by collective agreement. Seemingly traumatic experiences can be crucial to creating a shift and moving something towards a new balance not yet understood. Always put the intelligence of the land and situation above your own interpretation or need to be of service. And always ask permission before you do anything. If you get a response that everything is as it should be, honor it and leave things alone. Say hello, acknowledge the greater wisdom, and leave it at that.

If however you receive clear messages about something needed, then proceed according to your instructions. It is important to have your own set of tools, signs, ways of communicating, and specialties. The wisdom of the land will use your strengths so be clear about what you offer. For example, some are good at soul retrieval, some at singing, some at working with tobacco, some at working with specific allies including the four elements. So listen well, do what you are told to do, keep it simple, and never be attached to the outcome.

Sometimes it is helpful to have a set of personal signs for communicating and listening. You indicate what signs you will use and many of you already have a set of signs or symbols for this kind of work. Here are a few suggestions:

— The use of color, green light means yes, red light means no.
— Temperature, cool versus warm.
— Light intensity.
— Changes in your own body sensations.
— Working with winds and breezes.
— Smells.
— Certain allies showing up, a tap on the shoulder, a sensation behind the eyes.
— Acknowledging personal matching patterns.

Often you are drawn to working with an event or a location because of a matching pattern. On the one hand, it would make you more sensitive to what is needed, on the other hand, you could easily lose your neutrality as the trauma or disruption triggers something in your own personal history. This is actually likely to happen more often that not as it is almost natural to be drawn in to a circumstance that would promote some personal growth experience whenever possible. When this happens, acknowledge the personal trigger and take responsibility for your reactions. Be careful not to project your own process onto the land or onto others you may be working with. In this way you can still come from a place of neutrality while acknowledging that there may be a healing experience going on inside yourself at the same time. How do you know when you have hit a matching pattern? You lose your neutrality to judgment and attachment and feel emotions such as anger, grief, or despondency way beyond the situation you are working with. Acknowledge it as yours, have gratitude for the opportunity, and as much as is possible go back to working from a place of neutrality.

Protection

Whenever you step across the threshold between the physical and spirit world it is a good idea to have some protection around you either from one of your allies, something you visualize, or the use of a protective substance or object, such as smudging with tobacco or sage or carrying a special stone in your pocket. In this way you can keep your intuition and listening open without the fear of taking something on. Always ask for help with protection and always give thanks for the protection you receive. In the same discussion, it is almost always useful to clean yourself off with a clearing agent such as the smudge of sage, cedar, or tobacco, or by running a flourite crystal or other stone over yourself after doing this kind of work. Shamanic hygiene is part of good boundaries and helps with opening and closing a process from the place of integrity.

How do you know when the work is done?

This is perhaps the most challenging part of any process. You may rarely get a clear message that the "work" is done. It is however important that your portion of the "work" be complete. Whether it is a few minutes, several hours, a full day or more, remember that closing or completing is equally as important as initiating the process. This should always include saying thank you and releasing the allies you have called upon to help. There should also be a marker to release the container for the work and communication, something to mark that you are complete. You can use a drum, some sage to clear, or do some rattling or anything that says, "We're done." Do not worry about being perfect. Use you signs to know how much to do. If you are working in a group remember that everyone has something different to offer and there could be as many approaches and messages from the land as there are people involved. Don't let the ego compare, compete, be right, or need to control. There will always be something left to do at some point. However, if you get your personality out of the way and trust the higher wisdom and intelligence of the land, you cannot go wrong.

Using a Surrogate.

You can always work remotely on any situation or area using a surrogate. A surrogate can be anything from your own hand to an object such as a stone or something more symbolic. Set the intention for the object to symbolize and be a surrogate for what you wish to communicate with and it will be so. Remote work can be just as potent as being in location and equally as powerful. You would use the same protocol of saying hello, asking, listening, getting permission and help, doing what you are told, and closing.

Remember we are here to bless and be blessed. So be a blessing!

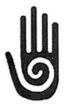

The Society of Shamanic Practitioners

THE SOCIETY OF SHAMANIC PRACTITIONERS (SSP) is an alliance of people deeply committed to the re-emergence of shamanic practices that promote healthy individuals and viable communities.

The Society is a not-for-profit public benefit corporation whose goal is to support the re-emergence of shamanism into modern, western culture. While many other shamanic organizations seek to document and learn from what has been done in the past, the Society is focused on the here and now and is interested in documenting how shamanism is changing and how it is being used as it interfaces with the twenty-first century world.

Society for Shamanic Practitioners
2300 Eighth Street, Olivenhain, California, USA 92024
www.shamansociety.org

AUTHORS

PAMELA ALBEE CCHT, CHI, RC is a registered counselor, certified clinical cypnotherapist, certified hypnotherapy instructor for the American Council of Hypnotist Examiners, and director of Stepping Stones Education Continuing Education Programs. She also has training in healing touch, emotional freedom techniques, and spiritual wellness.

CECILE CARSON, MD is a clinical associate professor of medicine and psychiatry at the University of Rochester Medical Center, Rochester, NY. An internist and counselor, she has focused her work over the past several decades on the mind-body-spirit interface in teaching and clinical care. She respects the endless variety of forms the healing process can take, and has explored and integrated a number of them: spiritual healing, hypnosis, neurolinguistic programming, therapeutic recreation, psychodrama, and dreamwork. Her extensive shamanic training with the FSS began in 1986 and included the Basic Workshop, 2-Week Intensive, Shamanic Counseling, Soul Retrieval, and the 3-Year East Coast Program. She also trained with a Romani *choviano*.

TOM COWAN, PHD is a shamanic practitioner specializing in Celtic visionary and healing techniques. He combines universal core shamanism with traditional European spirit lore to create spiritual practices that can heal and enrich one's own life and the lives of others. He is an internationally respected teacher, author, lecturer, and tour leader. He has taught training programs in England, Austria, Germany, Switzerland, Slovakia and Italy. Tom received a doctorate in history from St. Louis University. He has studied extensively with and taught for the Foundation for Shamanic Studies. Tom is the author of *Yearning for The Wind: Celtic Reflections on Nature and the Soul*, *Fire in the Head: Shamanism and The Celtic Spirit*, *Shamanism as a Spiritual Practice for Daily Life*, *The Pocket Guide to Shamanism*, *The Book of Seance*, *The Way of the Saints: Prayers, Practices, and Meditations* and *Wending Your Way: A New Version of the Old English Rune Poem*.

BONNIE J HORRIGAN is an artist, author, publisher, and executive who has been involved in shamanic study and mysticism since the early 1980s. The author of two books: *Red Moon Passage* (Harmony, 1996) and *Voices of Integrative Medicine: Conversations and Encounters* (Elsevier Science, 2003), she was the founding publisher of

Alternative Therapies in Health and Medicine, a breakthrough medical journal examining alternative and cross-cultural healing practices and the relationship of the human spirit to health and healing. She guided that journal to international acclaim for ten years. During that same time, while she was the president of InnoVision Communications, she helped launch the Shamanism and Medicine conference series with Alan Davis, MD, PhD. Bonnie helped to found the Society of Shamanic Practitioners with Alan Davis and Sandra Ingerman in the summer and fall of 2003. She now serves as editorial director for *EXPLORE: The Journal of Science and Healing*.

SANDRA INGERMAN, MA is the author of *Soul Retrieval: Mending the Fragmented Self* (Harper San Francisco 1991), *Welcome Home: Following Your Soul's Journey Home* (Harper San Francisco 1994), *A Fall to Grace* (Moon Tree Rising Productions 1997), and *Medicine for the Earth* (Three Rivers Press 2001). She is also the author of *The Beginner's Guide to Shamanic Journeying* and The Soul Retrieval Journey lecture programs and the book and CD program *Shamanic Journeying: A Beginner's Guide* produced by Sounds True. Sandra has an MA in Counseling Psychology from the California Institute of Integral Studies. She teaches workshops on shamanism around the world and was formerly the educational director of the Foundation for Shamanic Studies directed by Michael Harner. Sandra is recognized for bridging ancient cross-cultural healing methods into our modern day culture to address the needs of our times. Sandra is a licensed marriage and family therapist and professional mental health counselor in the state of New Mexico.

LORA JANSSON has been a shamanic practitioner and teacher for more than a decade. Shamanic work is her life, and she knows it is unique to each individual. She founded The Star Gazer Shamanic Moon Bear Project which organizes shamanic workers from all over the world to work for Moon Bears rescued from "bear farms" by Animals Asia Foundation (www.animalsasia.org).

ANA LARRAMENDI is a shamanic practitioner, teacher, minister, vision quest leader, and ceremonialist who has been studying and practicing shamanism since 1989. She is an initiated mesa carrier in the Inka tradition, a member of The Foundation for Shamanic Studies, and a founding member of the Society of Shamanic Practitioners. Ana has been a lecturer for the University of Wisconsin Medical School, and the Madison Area Technical College. Her ministerial service includes working with prisoners at the Prairie Du Chien Correctional Institute, hospital visitations, working with the dying, presiding over memorial services, officiating weddings, and supporting community ceremonies. Ana has a full-time practice working privately with clients for personal healing as well as doing land and space clearings.

CAROL PROUDFOOT-EDGAR has been studying and teaching shamanism for 20 years; prior to that she was a psychologist at the University of California, Santa Cruz. Twelve years ago she helped found the nonprofit organization Shamanic Circles. She has worked with a group of women physicians for 11 years to integrate shamanism and contemporary medical practice. Carol continues her work with a Clan of BearWomen that came into formal existence 16 years ago, and she has been teaching in the University of San Francisco Medical School's Integrative Medical Program. In the early 90's, she joined with Paul Rebillot to develop a paradigm regarding the evolution of the self that would integrate shamanism and Gestalt psychology. Out of this collaboration, Carol developed a *Medicine Wheel Handbook* that guides one through interrelationship between the personal and the transpersonal. Carol and her shamanic work are featured in Beverly Engel's book, *Women Encircling the Earth*, while her poetry and stories appear in a number of books and magazines. She has also produced two CDs containing healing songs that came to her from the spirits. Her writings and videos of her work with the National Geographic Society are available at her website : www.shamanicvisions.com.

JOSÉ LUIS STEVENS, PHD is the president and co-founder (with wife Lena) of Power Path Seminars, an international school and consulting firm dedicated to the study and application of shamanism and indigenous wisdom to business and everyday life. José completed a ten-year apprenticeship with a Huichol Maracame in the Sierras of Central Mexico. In addition, he is studying intensively with Shipibo in the Peruvian Amazon and with Pacos in the Andes in Peru. In 1983 he completed his doctoral dissertation at the California Institute of Integral Studies focusing on the interface between shamanism and western psychological counseling. Since then he has studied cross-cultural shamanism around the world to distill the core elements of shamanic healing and practice. He is the author of ten books and numerous articles including *The Power Path, Secrets of Shamanism: How to Tap the Spirit Power Within, Transforming Your Dragons*, and *Praying with Power*.

LENA STEVENS is an internationally known teacher and shamanic practitioner. She apprenticed for ten years with a Huichol shaman from Mexico and has studied cross-cultural shamanic healing from numerous traditions including those from the Amazon basin, Native North America, Northern Europe, and Siberia. One of her specialties is the woven song tradition of the Shipibo tribe in the Peruvian Amazon, the singing of Icaros or healing songs. Lena is the co-author of the *Secrets of Shamanism: How to Tap the Spirit Power Within* and a contributor to The Power Path.